double trouble

Twins and How to Survive Them

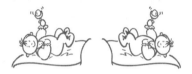

EMMA MAHONY

(with chapter cartoon illustrations
by Jonathan Pugh)

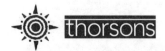
thorsons

Thorsons
An Imprint of HarperCollins*Publishers*
77–85 Fulham Palace Road
Hammersmith, London W6 8JB

The website address is:
www.thorsonselement.com

and *Thorsons* are trademarks of
HarperCollins*Publishers* Limited

Published by Thorsons 2003

7

© Emma Mahony 2003

A catalogue record of this book
is available from the British Library

ISBN-13   978-0-00-715398-5
ISBN-10   0-00-715398-8

Chapter Cartoon Illustrations by Jonathan Pugh

Printed and bound in Great Britain by
Clays Ltd, St Ives plc

This book is proudly printed on paper which contains wood
from well-managed forests, certified in accordance with
the rules of the Forest Stewardship Council.
For more information about FSC,
please visit www.fsc.org

Mixed Sources
Product group from well-managed
forests and other controlled sources
www.fsc.org Cert no. SW-COC-1806
© 1996 Forest Stewardship Council

FSC

For my twin brother and Olympic hero,
Dominic

Ten Great Things About Twins

1. You have an instant family – just add milk.
2. If you get fed up with one, you always have the other.
3. Nobody asks you whether you are going to have any more children (for a year, at least).
4. You never feel guilty about getting more help.
5. You get to eat 4,000 calories a day when breastfeeding (that's a tub of Häagen-Dazs and a pint of Guinness for lunch).
6. Twins start giggling at each other as soon as they can smile.
7. You make proper use of 'buy one get one free' offers at the supermarket.
8. You only have one birthday party to organize every year.
9. You become a local celebrity in the park and playground.
10. Your twins will turn out to be more confident, supportive, innovative, substantial, self-knowing, sought-after and giving than the average singleton.*

(* See *The Joy of Twins* in Further Reading at the back of the book.)

Contents

Acknowledgements

I would like to thank all those who shared their stories and wisdom within *Double Trouble*, and particularly those who read all or part of the manuscript before it was deemed fit for public consumption: my husband Adam, my mother and father, my midwives Annie Francis and Mary Cronk MBE, my agent Lesley Shaw, my publisher Wanda Whiteley and her sister with twins, Miranda, my editor Michele Turney, friends and colleagues Paul Richardson, Lisa Collins, Portia Colwell, Emma Mager, Susan Johnson, Victoria Pyman and Claire Pridham. Thanks also to the readers from the Wandsworth Twins Club – Susie Boone, Tamsin Cromwell and Megan Landon – and our au pair, Andrea Stehlíková.

Last but not least, the junior members of the band: my five-year-old Humphrey, who shared his room with my computer, and forced me to sing tuneless lullabies while I tapped away in the evening, and my adorable terrible twins Michael and Millie, who made the whole book possible (and impossible), as well as adding hundreds of zzzzzzzzzzzzzs and 88888888888888s into the text. Thanks guys.

Introduction

Welcome to the club. If you are reading this because you have just learnt that you are expecting twins, sit down. It may be your last chance. Whether you got to this point through good old genetic probability or, like a growing number, via the magic of IVF, congratulations! You are one of the most blessed people on the planet. Twins are the greatest gift in the world. I should know, because I am one. And I've never once had to worry about being the only person at my birthday party, because I've always had my brother there. And now I am doubly blessed, a twin who's had twins. What more could a woman want (okay, a career, a little more money, a husband who thinks you're Kylie, a flatter stomach – oops, sorry).

If you're reading this and you've already got twins, well done! You've made it back into the real world. You've made it into a shop, fully dressed (or did you buy this online, like most twin mothers?) And there's more good news. Like it or not, you have just become a lifetime member of the most inclusive club in the world. The twins club is a club where you will never again be stuck for conversation. From now on, you will have enough stories to entertain the oldest of grannies and the youngest of Teletubbies fans. You will discover the universal truth that everyone, old and young, loves twins. And the worse the stories are, the more they love them.

This is useful information to absorb now, because there will come a day when you feel like 'putting the twins out with the rubbish' (to paraphrase a comment from a three-year-old sibling). At that moment, you know you can load the babies into the double buggy and someone, somewhere, will stop you and say 'Are they twins? Aren't they gorgeous! Well, you *have* got your hands full.' And as you nod back in agreement, you will find all those frustrated feelings melt away. It's a funny thing, motherhood.

But for you pregnant women, that's all way, way into the future. Right now, all you care about is whether you will find any jeans to fit you in the last month and whether your husband will still love you when he can no longer fit in the bed. So, you've got the book in your hands, what are you waiting for? Now all you need is a box of chocolates ('eating for three' excuse) and a nice cup of raspberry leaf tea (if 'nice' and 'raspberry leaf tea' can sit in the same sentence) to settle down and prepare for the onslaught. I won't keep you too long – I know about pregnancy and attention spans, and **I will make any important stuff stand out in bold so you don't have to try too hard to remember it.**

For those who already have their twins, I hope this book will help you buy at least one good double buggy or learn a few tricks about how to stop the little angels crying. Or if you are a man reading this and have already got this far, feel free to skip straight to Chapter 12, 'The Fourth Trimester' and read the bit about Sex after Birth. I promise not to tell. Of course, as a woman who forgot to pack a proper hospital bag and brought her twins home wrapped in the midwives' scarves, I can't pretend to be an authority on everything. Because I know I don't have all the answers, I have canvassed dozens of other twin mothers who do.

This is a book that has been waiting to be written since I first started fighting my brother for a little more space in the cramped conditions of my mother's stomach. Because I am writing about twins from the perspective of being one, I feel at liberty to be a little more risqué on the subject than most. With the 'Double Trouble' column that has been running for the past two years in *The Times*, I have weathered enough 'shocked' and 'disgusted' letters from older mothers to know that times have changed. Modern mothers need a laugh every now and then to sustain them through the early years, and none more so than twin mums. It is therefore no coincidence that I have enlisted the help of my talented friend at *The Times*, Johnny Pugh, to remind us of this every now and then. I feel happiest when working in a team of two (that twin thing again), and Johnny's insights into family life have been earned at the coalface of fatherhood.

Are there any messages to take from this book? Only two, surprisingly. The first is that you are a lucky, lucky person. The second is that your life will never be the same again. Different, better, but never the same. Welcome to the world of twins. I shall go now, and tread lightly for fear of waking mine up...

'Your children are not your children
They are the sons and daughters of life's longing for itself'

KAHLIL GIBRAN,
THE PROPHET, 1923

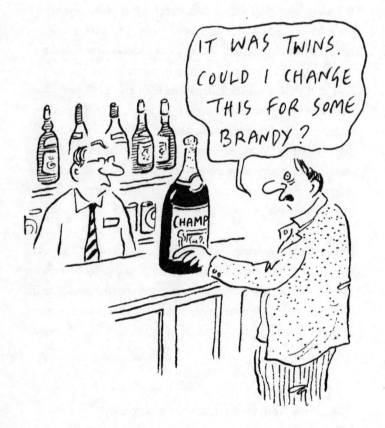

ONE

Twinshock

It may have taken an American to coin the phrase 'twin-shock', but the sensation is felt the world over. There is no easy way to learn the news. It helps if your hand is being held by the man responsible (more possible if it's your first pregnancy, less probable if it's your second) or if you have a sympathetic sonographer doing the scan, but, once the word is out, the impact will take your breath away. Being told that you are expecting twins will resonate deep in your psyche, announcing that your life is about to change for good.

For this reason, sonographers doing the ultrasound often try and fudge the moment with comments such as: 'There seems to be two. Let me check if there's three' (this happened to Joanne Pinkess, who heaved a huge sigh of relief that it was not triplets). Another girlfriend, Heather, was asked: 'Would you like the good news or the bad news?' With four children already, she asked for both. 'The good news is that everything is fine,' said the scanner, 'the bad news is that you're expecting twins.'

The other approach is to push the responsibility for the diagnosis on to you. The sonographer scanning Judy Collins, with her husband Jim beside her, turned to poor Jim to announce the news. 'What's the first thing you can see?' she asked, turning the screen to the husband. Jim saw two blobs, so said 'two eyes?' 'No,' she corrected him, 'two babies.'

However you learn, try and hang on to that initial moment and build it into a story for later. Not only will you be asked dozens of times before your life is over, but your twins will have to recount the moment, too. If only I had a pound for every time I've had to retell the story of my mother going into labour, and the midwife calling over the doctor to ask 'Can you hear *two* heartbeats here?' Sadly for my father, he was in the pub. My, how times have changed.

Tears and light blasphemy

From the mothers I've asked, the most common response to the news they were expecting twins seems to be tears and light blasphemy. I had my three-year-old with me for the 12-week scan, and he was ramming a Thomas the Tank Engine train into my thigh while the sonographer slopped gel on my stomach and swirled the scanner over my paunch for a good five minutes before choosing her moment. 'Have you been experiencing anything unusual about this pregnancy?' she ventured. 'Oh, you know, a lot more tired than with the first,' I answered, preparing for a moan. 'Peep, peep,' squeaked Thomas at my knee. 'Well,' she continued in her best breezy voice 'there is something I have to tell you…' (a line that never goes down well with pregnant mothers). I sat up immediately, expecting the worst unmentionable diagnosis. 'You've got two babies in there!' she blurted. 'Ohmygod, Ohmygod, Ohmygod,' I answered.

A few minutes later, as she helped me out of the darkened scanning room, I felt twice as pregnant as before I went in, suddenly more sow than goddess. I was directed around the corner for the next NHS appointment and for my next shock – that the hospital had no room for me. Even if they had told me that there was a Stannah Stairlift and a red carpet up to the delivery room, I would have burst into tears at that point. It was as if the initial shock was receding and reality setting in. I boo-hooed so loudly at the reception desk that a flurry of doctors suddenly poked their heads out of their doors and a kind female doctor came out to investigate. Seeing the waiting room full of anxious pregnant mothers, now massaging their bumps a little more nervously, she whisked me into her office. There she explained the relative merits of all the local hospitals, from how new their maternity units were to how many beds they held, to reassure me that if I couldn't make it into my chosen Chelsea and Westminster there were others that would have me.

It was to be my first lesson about carrying twins and the National Health Service (make a noise to get help from anyone, blubbing loudly if necessary). I also learnt that from that day forward, and particularly when the twins were born, I was to be the entertainment for the waiting room.

Numb with no tears

Not everyone reacts with such drama. Triplet (heroine) mother Valerie Cormack had a variation on twinshock when she was told at her first scan. She sat in a daze at the news and described her reaction as 'horror and worry'.

'My first thought was "how will I manage this?", and my second thought was "where are we going to put them?" – our house isn't that big.' Valerie, 34, had her mother with her because her husband Andy was away on business. When she told Andy, his reaction more than made up for her state of numbness. 'He was thrilled. He said "Isn't it great! We've always wanted a family and now we've got three children!"' A week later, Valerie's fears began to subside and she started to feel happy about it.

Preparing the siblings

Just as there is no perfect time to deliver the news to an absent spouse, there is also no perfect time to prepare other children.

I had my three-year-old little boy to tell, who had been vaguely aware of the histrionics in obstetrics, but was really far more interested in his Brio engine. Rather than sit him down and Have The Talk, I decided to prep him whenever he brought up the subject. A colleague at work, both of whose parents were psychologists, warned me against The Talk.

Apparently, when she was little and her parents had tried to prepare her for the arrival of her brother, she had nodded all through their explanation of forthcoming family life. At the end, they asked if she had any questions. She replied earnestly: 'Mummy, will it have a head?'

When my son Humphrey showed any interest in my stomach, I would say proudly 'Mummy's got two babies in her tummy.' One day, as I was continuing to reinforce the message, he stuck out his stomach and said 'Humphrey's got two babies in there, too.'

I have to say that Humphrey's reaction was a little better than four-year-old Jake, the elder sibling of non-identical twin girls in Lewisham, south-east London. When Jake was taken along with his mother and father to the 12-week scan to share in the excitement of his new brother or sister, there were even more tears. 'It soon became obvious that the scanner was on to something,' said Paul, his father. 'The first we knew was when she turned to my wife and asked whether we had a history of twins in the family.' Jake asked his father what 'twins' meant. 'It's very special,' said Paul, in twinshock himself but choosing his words carefully, 'there's not going to be one baby, but two!' Jake promptly burst into tears, howling: 'But Daddy, I don't want two babies, I only want one.'

Telling the office

There is only one good rule when it comes to the office: tell them as late as you can get away with (which won't be *that* late on with twins). If you are someone who likes to be the centre of attention, then blurt the news out as early as you like. However, the rest of us will find a twin pregnancy a rude awakening. It is the equivalent of dressing up in a clown out-fit and wearing a big red nose.

From the moment everyone knows in the office, you will spend the rest of the run-up to maternity leave answering questions on whether you have chosen names, found out sexes, or, worse, how cousin Ethelberga had twins and was committed to a psychiatric hospital shortly after. Nobody will be interested in how well you gave that presentation, or took the minutes of the meeting, only in the gusset of your elasticated trousers. If you want to be taken seriously, don't let on until the most tactless person finally asks. Then you know that you can hide it no longer, and the truth will out. By then you will have your handbag ready on the desk to swat the next person who makes a bad joke. Go in hard to deflect the more cautious jokers out there.

Scans, scans, scans

It is well worth making friends with the staff in the ultra-sound department because you are going to see a lot of them by the end of your pregnancy. A box of Quality Street never goes amiss. Once they have spotted twins, they'll probably expect you to come in every fortnight after 28 weeks (just when you don't feel like moving far), as well as having the usual 12-week and 20-week scans. What they are checking for is how the twins are growing and whether they are lying head down or head up, which will make a difference to the birth. Particularly with identical twins sharing a placenta, they are looking to see whether one of the twins takes the lion's share of the food (twin-to-twin transfusion, a great name for a '70s rock band). In the unlikely event that there is a dominant and greedy twin, they may suggest delivering the babies ahead of time. One friend of mine was told by the sonographer that she could continue with her identical-twin pregnancy without being induced because the twins were exactly the same weight at around 5lb. When born, one twin was over 7lb – two pounds heavier than the original estimate. It turns out that they measured the same twin twice.

So, scans may look like a precise science, but they aren't. Sexes are wrongly reported, anomalies not picked up, and suggested birth weights are often wildly inaccurate. All this human error is further confused by giving you probability equations to do in your head, when everyone knows pregnant women can't do maths.

'Excuse me, is a one in 500 chance in the Nuchal Translucency test a good result or a bad result? Does that mean that if I have 499 children, the 500th may have Down's syndrome? Or will it mean that one of my twins will have it, and the next 199 sets of twins I produce won't? But won't I be given another nonsensical probability equation at those subsequent pregnancies? Why can't someone just say "yes" or "no"? Anyway, we've already decided that if we do have a Down's baby we are carrying on with the pregnancy. Which begs the question: why are you scanning me in the first place?' This is what I would like to have said to the sonographer. Instead, like thousands of pregnant women, I just nodded and felt a little scared.

If you do feel anxious at the prospect of a scan, take your partner, mother or girlfriend with you. They can listen while you feel fearful. And, if you are unhappy about any scan diagnosis, ask to be scanned again by the head of ultrasound in the hospital. Scans are so often wrong, they are not worth losing sleep over.

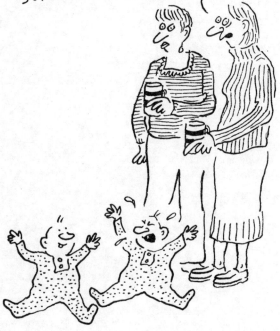

TWO

What Flavour Are They?

Okay, I promised in the Introduction that I wouldn't befuddle you with words like 'monochorionic' and 'dizygosity', but the time has come to get the dictionary out. You may as well get a handle on what flavour your twins are, because throughout your and their life, plenty of people will try to tell you differently. You will be amazed at how many intelligent people were obviously sound asleep during their biology lessons.

All twins are identical (not)

People desperately want to believe that all twins are alike. There is some deep-seated desire in the human soul that needs to believe this. It is not a rational thing. Perhaps it is steeped in our ancient tribal belief that we must hunt in identical pairs. Or maybe it's a more modern, narcissistic view that when we die, a clone of ourselves will continue to carry on our important genetic heritage and be available for medical science when needed. Some people will even argue with you that 'your twins are not proper twins' unless they are identical.

This means that if you have fraternal (non-identical) twins (another misnomer to make all twins sound like brothers), you will often be asked 'are they identical?' Even if you have boy and girl twins, and the girl is standing in pigtails and a dress and the boy is brushing mud off his football kit, the same stupid question will be asked again and again. And don't be fooled by the intelligence of the interlocutor. My headmaster asked my brother and I the very question in front of the whole school when we went up to receive two different awards at an end-of-term ceremony. In this instance I refrained from my stock answer ('No, he has a willy and I don't'). However, I highly recommend this one for closing the subject quickly.

If you have non-identical girl twins, or non-identical boy twins, you may need to engage in a brief biology lesson, particularly when your answer of 'No' will be met by disbelief. 'No, they came from two separate eggs and two separate sperms,' is usually pitched at the right level. Most people's eyes will glaze over at the mention of zygosity.

The truth, however, is a little more complicated. And if you only read the following once in your life, it will give you some insight into why twins are so endlessly fascinating to the medical establishment.

Boy/Girl Twins

Girls and boys cannot be identical. Nobody mistakes a brother and sister for each other, so why do people mistake boy/girl twins? Statistics[1] show the national average for boy/girl twins to be 33 per cent of all fraternal twin births. Expect around 100 per cent of the population to ask you 'Why don't they look the same?' Women are more likely to have fraternal twins if there is any incidence of twins on their *mother's* side (not their father's).

Non-identical Girl/Girl or Boy/Boy twins

Statistics also show that 33 per cent of all non-identical twins are two-egg girl/girl combinations, and the other 33 per cent are two-egg boy/boy combinations. These twins will show the normal sibling differences in temperament, intelligence, social interests and choice of pop music. Unlike their identical counterparts, where studies have shown twins to co-operate more with each other, fraternals are, if anything, more competitive than other siblings. This is not a given – again it's back to temperament – but it is worth preparing for, especially in toddlerhood (where buying two identical ride-on cars will save you having to shout constantly 'SHARING, for God's sake!'). Competitiveness among twins is not that surprising when you consider they have to compete for everything from day one, from mother's milk to parental attention.

Nor should acquiring a competitive edge be considered a down-side. My twin brother went on to win a bronze medal at the Olympic Games in modern pentathlon (running, riding, swimming, fencing and shooting). I am sure he honed his skills in the back garden while running away from me in my nurse's outfit.

Identical twins

Identical twins are sometimes described as 'a freak of nature', because there is no genetic reason for producing them. Unlike fraternal twins, that follow the mother's hereditary line, identical twins are theoretically a one-off occurring in one in every three twin births.

Not all 20-week scans, when you can tell the sex of the babies, can diagnose for sure whether the twins are identical or not. Sometimes with identical twins the egg splits later in the pregnancy, between day 7 and 14, resulting in separate placentas and separate sacs. To confuse matters further, non-identical twins can sometimes be misdiagnosed by ultrasound scans when their two placentas have fused into one.

There are now two types of test done at birth to confirm for sure whether the twins are identical or not – a blood test to compare blood factors, and the more recent DNA finger-printing. Parents of identical twins usually want to know the results, not only to establish their birthright, but also for medical reasons. If one child shows susceptibility to allergy, asthma or any childhood illnesses, they will be better informed to protect the other.

One good thing about identical twins is that when people ask you: 'Are they identical?' You can answer 'Yes!' (and so can your twins). However, be prepared for fresh idiocy. Caroline Watton, who has identical twin girls, was stopped by an old lady in the supermarket as she was pushing the girls around in a trolley. 'Ooh, aren't they sweet!' cooed the old woman. 'Are they identical?' Before Caroline could answer 'Yes', the woman contradicted her. 'Of course they're not!' she said. 'Look, one's fast asleep and the other's awake.' The nation's biology teachers have a lot to answer for.

Just to confuse you further...

As well as the simple and straightforward combinations, there are small differences that will really make you confused. I don't recommend you venture into conversation with any old women in the supermarket about the following subjects.

Mirror-image twins

About a third of all identical twins are 'mirror-image twins'. If the one egg that splits does so later in the pregnancy, after the seventh day, then sometimes the twins have mirror-image traits – such as one is left-handed, the other right-handed. As they grow, you might notice one sprouting a tooth on one side, while the other does so on the other side, or different hair whorls curling in opposite ways. No-one is exactly sure what causes this effect, but it all adds to the mythology surrounding identical twins.

Identical twins who don't look alike

Because some identicals share a placenta, and don't always have equal access to the nutrition because of how they are lying in the womb, they may have quite different birth weights. The weight soon equalizes after birth, however, but the changes in the shape of the face or bodily difference may stay for life. Identicals may also have slightly different hair colour and birthmarks.

Twins that result from superfecundation

Superfecundation describes the fertilization of two eggs after two or more bouts of sex during the same menstrual cycle. Given the small window of ovulation and the short lifetime of a sperm, these bouts of sex have to take place quite close together. Very interesting. Could this be you? (unlikely if you have any other children in the house).

Superfecundation gives rise to the possibility of twins with two different fathers, for women who might wave their husbands off to work and then open the back door to the milkman. Rare incidents of mixed-race twins where one baby is born black and the other white can also happen in normal twin conception with the same father, as in the case of the twins Karen and Cheryl Grant from Essex, now 19.

IVF or natural? Who cares?

I've included the question of whether your twins are 'IVF' or 'natural' because you'd be amazed at how many people think it is their business. You have probably already been asked this, usually by Ms Nosey Parker.

My view, whether you conceived with the help of IVF or not, is to tell people a lie. Anyone tactless enough to ask deserves to be led astray. As long as those who conceived naturally are quick to answer 'naturally', as if there is something inherently better about this answer, then people will continue to ask. Perhaps you could ask a question back to Ms Parker, such as 'What is IVF exactly?' and then nod interestedly as she attempts to explain. Then ask her, regardless of whether she's had children or not, whether she's had IVF herself, because she seems such an authority on the subject.

Men and the assisted conception business

When my husband told a West Indian client that his wife was expecting twins, the client slapped him on the back and shouted, 'Congratulations! Mon, you shoot with double barrel, never miss – Bam! Bam!' The Jamaican summed up the view that all men secretly share – that twins are an expression of a man's (not a woman's) fertility. I haven't met a single father of twins who hasn't puffed up his chest when remembering his own important walk-on part in the twin drama.

Of course, all women know that this Woody Allen view of sperm is ridiculous, and that all sorts of complicated factors are involved to make conception possible. However, there is no harm in encouraging this virile fantasy (and if that means suppressing the information that they are IVF, just carry on lying) because a swaggering partner in the early days is more likely to be a helpful one later on. All women know this instinctively, so you don't really need to be told.

The IVF twin mix-up stories

The 'mix-up-in-the-lab' story is recycled again and again whenever the latest fertility scare happens. This is a variation on every woman's irrational fear that her baby will be switched by mistake when the nurses are chatting abstractedly over a cup of tea. This fear is as old as the hills. My mother admits to being so scared by it that she insisted on having a home birth for her first born, back in 1961. When my 11lb (ouch!) big brother finally appeared, I think few would have mixed him up with some 5lb weakling.

There are three twin mix-up tales in the IVF history books. The first was when a white mother gave birth to black twins in the summer of 2002 here in Britain. The sperm was wrongly mixed with the woman's eggs after a laboratory error in an NHS clinic, and the legal outcome determining who are the parents has yet to be settled.

The other two happened elsewhere in the world. The first was in 1993 in Holland where twin boys, one white and one black, were born to Willem and Wilma Stuart after two samples of sperm became accidentally mixed before being used to fertilize Wilma's eggs. The biological father made no attempts to gain custody of his twin, but the family keeps in touch in the event that his biological son may want to meet him one day.

The second case happened in 1998 in New York when two lots of embryos were mixed and both women, Donna Fasano and Deborah Rogers, were implanted with what they took to be their own embryos. Only one of the pregnancies turned out to be successful, and the mother had one black and one white twin. There followed a difficult legal battle, leading to the black twin being handed over to his biological mother. Despite the recrimination between the parents and the hospital, the now four-year-old twins still visit each other.

Natural or not so natural?

The folic acid factor

New research[2] also suggests that women who take folic acid are nearly twice as likely to give birth to twins as women who do not. A higher rate of twin births in relation to folic acid was first noticed in an earlier Hungarian trial. The recent Swedish research team examined Swedish records since 1994. The scientists found that among 2,569 women who had used folic acid supplements, the rate of twin births was 2.8 per cent – nearly double the normal level of 1.5 per cent. They are unsure why folic acid might be responsible for producing more twins. It is possible that folic acid encourages multiple ovulations or the implantation of more than one egg. It might also prevent the spontaneous abortion of one or more foetuses occurring in women who do not take folic acid.

The official advice is still for women to take 400mcg of supplemented folic acid before conception and for the first three months of pregnancy (see also www.hsis.org – Health Supplements Information Service).

I took 12 times the recommended dosage because my first baby was born with a cleft lip and palate, so I read the study with interest. But, then again, I also fell into all of the other categories that made me more likely to have twins: I was over 35, taller and heavier (charming) than your average British mother, a twin myself who had already had one child.

TWIN PREGNANCY VITAL STATISTICS[3]

Natural conception:

- The chance of having twins rises steadily as the mother gets older.
- The peak age is 35 to 39 for European women.
- Women are more likely to have twins the more children they have, independent of their age.
- Fraternal or non-identical twins are more common if there is a presence of twins on the mother's side of the family (contrary to popular opinion, the father's side makes no difference).
- Identical twins are random and occur in one in three of all twin births (although scientists are still trying to explain why they occur more in some families).
- You can insure against the extra cost of having twins before your 14th week of pregnancy, providing you are not having IVF treatment and have yet to be scanned by your doctor. At the time of going to print, insurance company Marcus Hearn (0207 739 3444) will pay out £1,000 for a minimum premium of £42.

Assisted conception:

- Since the very first test-tube baby Louise Brown was born in Britain in 1978, in vitro fertilization now accounts for around 8,000 babies born every year in Britain.
- One in four IVF pregnancies results in twins.
- The number of triplet births has risen from 91 in 1980 to 262 in 2002.
- The number of twin births has grown from 6,400 in 1980 to 8,500 in 2002.
- In Britain alone, the number of cycles of treatment has risen from 28,000 in 1991 to 44,000 in 2002.
- A quarter of infertile couples succeed with IVF.

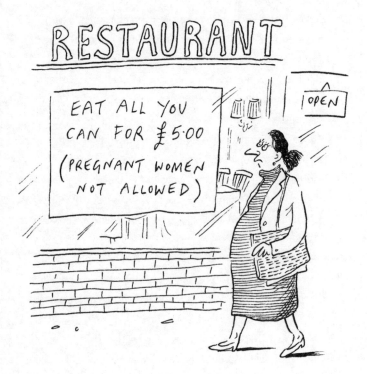

THREE

Eating and Exercising for Three

Make no mistake: one good thing about a twin pregnancy is that you get to eat a lot, and most of the weight will go on the babies. All of us who have had guilt issues surrounding food can now look forward to nine months of bingeing, and even longer if you hope to breastfeed. **For a twin pregnancy, you are not only invited to eat one-and-a-half times more than for a singleton pregnancy, it is practically a responsibility.** [1]

There is also enough evidence now to support the welcome news that in a twin pregnancy there is a direct correlation between higher maternal weight gain and better birth outcomes.[2] So, what are you waiting for? Order that Fortnum & Mason hamper now. This should be the rekindling of a long love affair with food.

During my own twin pregnancy, which was remarkably trouble-free and ran the whole course to term at 40 weeks, I went food mad. I decided to allow myself absolutely no restrictions on the amount of food I ate, and arrived at work having visited the deli with two plastic bags from the greengrocer and the baker en route. For all my no-holds-barred approach, I was very picky about the type and quality of food I ate. In my first pregnancy, I had put on a lot of weight by eating badly, pretending that my penchant for crisps, cider and Maltesers was a craving. It took me 18 months to shift the excess stone (or two).

Second time around, I had learnt my lesson about office vending machines and was careful about the type of food I ate. I would bring in as much fruit and raw veg as I could carry – carrots, cucumber, tomatoes, cauliflower, apples, bananas and grapes. Added to this would be a mixture of cheese, quiches and whatever else shouted 'eat me!' from the deli that day. Should anyone ever question you on the size of that cheese sandwich you are about to put in your mouth, just remind them that you are 'eating for three'.

The first three months

The most important eating time is the first three months, when the babies are, literally, being created. This is when the nutrient factor is most crucial. Do not fret if you are among the many twin mothers who suffer from **morning sickness.** Multiple mothers tend to have a higher level of pregnancy hormone in their blood so they experience more nausea and vomiting than their singleton friends.[3] Paradoxically, if you suffer from bad morning sickness and can't keep the food down for long, this won't affect the babies' eventual birth weight. It's the nutrients they are after, not the fat. And they will take the nutrients from your own body's supply if you don't provide them (get used to it, it goes with the territory). Mothers with morning sickness should be heartened by the research showing that sufferers have babies with better overall outcomes. Studies suggest that vomiting may stimulate early placental growth.

If you feel tired and sluggish in the first three months, but not nauseous, remember that your body is making two babies *and* extra blood volume. For twins you can expect a 75 per cent increase in your blood volume (for triplets there's a 100 per cent increase).[4] Add to this the fact that a mother pregnant with twins can carry up to 20 pints of water more than a mother of a singleton during her pregnancy, and you can see why you have a perfect excuse to take to your bed at 8pm. Things will ease up in the second trimester, your metabolism will go into high gear, and the weight you gain will all go towards making healthy babies.

Just say 'no!' to the calorie counters

Personally, as a poor maths student, the calorie-counting view of the world has never appealed. It turns a sensuous experience, eating, into a tax return. Also, for twin pregnancies, I've noticed that the number of calories suggested by 'experts' varies wildly. In my own twin book library, the figures range from 2,700 calories to 3,500 per day. However, if calorie counting helps you to feel in control, aim for somewhere in the middle.

My main beef against calorie counting is that it puts you in the frame of mind of dieting, which is the wrong thing to do when pregnant. Also, anything that limits your intake of food ('I've eaten my 3,500 calories today, I should stop now and just drink water') should be avoided. This is your time for growing the babies, so enjoy it. No other vices are possible in pregnancy (you may get away with lust for a few weeks, but the wolf whistles will disappear by that last trimester), so you may as well indulge in gluttony.

One mother of twins was told by a nurse that she was gaining weight too fast and should stop drinking milk. When she told her husband, he opened the fridge door, took out a two-pint carton and handed it to her. She drank the whole lot on the spot. Don't listen to any jealous nurses or doctors on the subject. Listen to your body. If you are hungry, it is for a good reason.

Never weigh yourself during pregnancy

Another trick in pregnancy is to never ever weigh yourself. If the midwife wanted to weigh me at the checkup, I asked her to put it in kilos, and my mathematical dyslexia ensured that it stayed a mystery. I found the best place to put my scales was in the loft until the babies' first birthday. And if you plan to breastfeed for longer, chuck the scales out and buy some new ones when you are ready.

If, however, you are wedded to weight-gain issues, American charts suggest the following:

- By the 24th week of a twin pregnancy you should have gained double the number of pounds as a singleton mother – between 24 and 30lb.
- By the 37th week you should be around 50lb heavier than your normal weight.[5]

Use these figures only if they help you feel more comfortable about your weight gain.

Why tons of fruit and veg are a good idea

Recent research[6] also suggests that eating plenty of fruit and veg before and during pregnancy may protect against pre-eclampsia. This condition, which is a little more common in twin pregnancies and often appears in the final stages of pregnancy, is characterized by high blood pressure and swelling (my midwife always used to tell me 'if you can't get your wedding band off, call me'). Pre-eclampsia is a treatable but serious concern for pregnant mothers, and can sometimes necessitate an early delivery. It has to be monitored because, left untreated, it can eventually affect the function of liver and kidneys. Routine urine tests during pregnancy check for a type of protein which indicates pre-eclampsia.

New research shows that an underlying factor in pre-eclampsia is damage to blood vessels caused by destructive molecules called free radicals. In theory, upping the intake of nutrients that combat free-radical damage – such as vitamin C, found naturally in fruit and veg – may help to reduce the risk of pre-eclampsia. Another reason to gorge yourself at the greengrocers.

Why fish is also good

There is no dispute that well-fed women seem to make healthier babies with higher birth weights. What is news is recent research from Danish scientists reported in the *British Medical Journal* which suggests that women who eat a diet rich in fish are nearly four times less likely to give birth prematurely. Among 8,700 pregnant women surveyed, 7.1 per cent who never ate fish had a premature delivery, yet only 1.9 per cent of fish-eaters did. This is quite a significant finding for twin mothers, whose babies are usually assumed to be premature. So get baking that fish pie.

What can't I eat?

Raw fish, such as sushi, is to be avoided. It increases your risk of exposure to salmonella, parasites and hepatitis A infection that can damage your liver. Similarly, you should avoid **uncooked eggs** and **unpasteurized cheeses**. Finally, **peanuts** (which aren't actually nuts but beans) are still a controversial food item, because some experts believe that including them in your diet sensitizes the baby to peanut allergy. There is no definitive study to show this, but it's best to avoid them and err on the side of caution.

If you do eat or have already eaten any of the above by mistake, as I have during both my pregnancies, do not panic. Remember that you come from a long line of genetically-fit ancestors, and your pregnant forebears probably feasted happily on Stilton crawling with maggots and boiled boar's head.

What the experts say

Suzannah Olivier, author of *Eating for a Perfect Pregnancy* (Simon & Schuster Pocket Books) has the following advice to offer twin mothers:

'The important thing in any pregnancy, particularly a twin pregnancy, is to eat 'nutrient dense' food. Everything provides nutrients, bar sugar, which is empty calories and gives energy without providing nutrients.

'The other thing is to have more calories than normal. You are going to put on extra weight because of that extra placenta and amniotic fluid. For nutrient-dense food, think of half an avocado rather than extra butter on your bread.

'Remember, you need these nutrients for yourself as well as the baby in the post-natal stage. To get through those first six months, you need to build up your reserves. You are going to lose a lot of iron, zinc and essential fats in the last trimester and from the birth and the early months of breastfeeding.

'Food-wise, nuts – tree nuts such as almonds and walnuts – seeds, pulses and oily fish are all good. Zinc is found in any protein-rich food, like red meat.

'In the third trimester, zinc and essential fats are particularly important for growth. If there's not enough in the diet the baby will take it from the mother's reserves (a lot of postnatal depression may be linked in part to the mother's depletion of zinc and essential fatty acids). Good nutrients also help your own energy levels and stabilize your moods after birth. Often eczema in the mother while breastfeeding is triggered by not having enough essential fats. If you take linseed flax oil, it works very quickly to improve your condition.

'Two other key nutrients are calcium-rich foods and antioxidant-rich foods, found in fruit and veg. We tend to take a sledge-hammer approach to calcium and just drink milk (yoghurt is also good because it is predigested by bacteria), but there are swathes of people who are lactose intolerant. Many people don't realize that there is plenty of calcium and magnesium in green, leafy veg such as spinach, cabbage, pumpkin seeds, pine nuts and sunflower seeds. Raisins and dried apricots are also unexpected sources of calcium, magnesium, potassium and iron – all needed for bone health.

'Finally, I would strongly advise every mother pregnant with multiples to take a specially formulated **prenatal supplement** all through the pregnancy. You can buy them at any chemist, and it's never too late to start.'

Here is what four triplet (heroine) mothers ate during pregnancy to produce three healthy babies.

'I ate a lot of toast and Vegemite (my favourite), apples and cheese and lots of red meat (which I found pretty horrible!).'

Susi Gorbey, mother of Abigail, Lucille and Manon, went to 38 weeks with her triplets ('Don't let the doctors bully you into delivering early')

'I'm a vegetarian, and ate organic food as much as possible during my pregnancy. I ate plenty of fresh foods, but nausea restricted me a lot. I wanted to eat "comfort food" – pies, quiches, potatos, savoury carbohydrates. I avoided caffeine, alcohol, aspartame/phenylalanine as found in fizzy drinks.'

Tracy Alter, mother of Jake, Luke and Daniel

'I didn't change much of my diet during pregnancy as we eat a fairly healthy diet in any event. The only change was not drinking alcohol at all and starting every morning with a good breakfast that included flax seed – which I swear kept me extremely well throughout my pregnancy. I didn't really have a favourite food and didn't have any cravings.'

Marion Davies, mother of Thomas, Helen and Emma

'I was either sick or nauseous throughout my entire pregnancy, so ate a lot of whatever didn't come back up. I steered clear of complex carbohydrates. What I liked best was ice cubes!'

Alex Salmon, mother of Freddy, Lulu and Alexander

Exercise for the permanently tired

There is a lot to be said for keeping fit in pregnancy. Not running around sort of fit, but keeping moving sort of fit, as a preparation for labour. **Walking, swimming and yoga are all thoroughly recommended in both the early and late stages, and can be done right up to the day of delivery.**

Swimming is the best exercise for twin mothers towards the end, particularly if you are a member of a clean health club (pregnancy makes you notice the plasters on the bottom of the public pool). I loved the feeling of weightlessness as I took to the water, cupping my stomach and the babies as I slowly made my way up and down the pool. I even managed to escape buying a maternity swimming costume by wearing a black Lycra size 20 until the very end. Swimming is also good because it keeps your temperature stable in the water, increases blood flow and urine output, and reduces swelling. At the same time, it puts less stress on other parts of your body, particularly the uterus.

Yoga is also wonderful if you can find a pre-natal class locally, or a yoga teacher who can show you a few simple exercises to do. Pre-natal classes, as opposed to normal classes, also give you the opportunity to sit around chatting to other pregnant women while the yoga teacher reminds you to do your pelvic floor exercises.

Love your pelvic floor

The pelvic floor muscles are what your expanding babies are sitting on. They sit like a hammock supporting your internal organs, and withstand a lot of pressure during pregnancy. Regardless of whether you have elected for a Caesarean and are hoping to escape 'honeymoon sweet' (a myth, I'm afraid), **you need to learn to love your pelvic floor muscles. It is pregnancy, not birth, that stretches them, so nobody escapes.** If you don't learn to love them now, you may never set foot on a trampoline again, or survive a coughing fit without a dash to the loo. Take those Bangkok girls with ping-pong balls as your role models and 'squeeeeze!' (in the words of the heroine of Allison Pearson's hilarious novel *I Don't Know How She Does It* [7]).

Once a yoga teacher has helped you locate your pelvic floor, find a regular place to do your exercises, such as when sitting at the traffic lights. The only place I could remember was in the bath. Lying on my back, I would do the hold for 10 seconds, release for 10 seconds, hold for 9 seconds, release for 9 seconds, until the water went cold. Those without a yoga teacher can practise by sitting on the loo and holding back their pee intermittently.

Working out

As I have never set foot in a gym, I can't give any sensible advice on what exercises can and can't be done in later pregnancy. However, the actress Jane Seymour writes quite comprehensively about her workout regime before the birth of her twin boys Kris and Johnny. Without wishing to pour cold water on her efforts, her impressive gym activity is tempered by the fact that she did go into labour at 34 weeks after the onset of pre-eclampsia. (Her disappointment about being wheeled in for an emergency Caesarean, however, was offset by the surgeon's flattering remarks as she lay under the knife. In her book *Two at a Time* the surgeon is quoted as saying, 'Look at those abdominal muscles – good work, Jane. They look like the muscles of a 20-year-old.'[8] The following excerpt from her punishing schedule carries a warning that you may well feel tired just reading it:

'My workout stayed essentially the same between 28 weeks and 34 weeks with some important exceptions because of the irritable uterus episode I'd had at 28 weeks. I no longer warmed up on either the recumbent bike or the Stairmaster. I also used stretchy exercise bands instead of the weight machine, and I did exercises seated or lying down instead of standing. Gently, I kept up with my abdominal exercises, even though I had grown so large, although Dr Ross pointed out that if I had experienced pre-term labour, all abdominal exercises would have been out.'

Phew. Cup of raspberry leaf tea, anyone?

Obviously now is not the time to take up jogging, because there is nothing more uncomfortable than your stomach and boobs swinging up towards your face. But for those of you who were runners before your body was invaded, there is little reason why, with the blessing of your doctor or midwife, you can't carry on. In the Autumn issue of our twins club newsletter, we reported on a 33-year-old marathon runner who became pregnant with twins. After her first antenatal visit she cut down her running from 96 miles a week to around 66 miles, and eased off her pace. The twins grew at a normal rate and the mother stayed healthy, only giving up running three days before the birth. After a planned Caesarean at 36 weeks, she gave birth to twins weighing 4lb 14oz (2.2kg) and 5lb 1oz (2.3kg). Go girl.

Dealing with common complaints

Ranking in order of popularity, from the most popular complaint to the least popular, here are the most common symptoms that 50 twin mothers in our local south-west London area experienced in moderation during their pregnancy. The questionnaire did not include 'exhaustion' which was cited by everyone. Suggested remedies are in brackets next to the complaints.

- Backache (48% – yoga)
- Indigestion (42% – glug Gaviscon, which you can buy or get from your GP on free prescription in industrial sizes to alleviate symptoms)
- Sickness (34% – ice cubes, lemon juice and water mouthwashes, boiled sweets and ginger products such as tea and preserves, but not concentrated ginger capsules – all seem to help some but not others.)
- Swollen lower limbs (23% – swim or lie down)
- Swollen upper limbs (21% – swim or lie down)
- Higher blood pressure (5% – lie down and leave work)

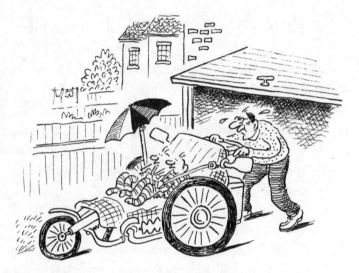

FOUR

I Shop, Therefore I Am

When I interviewed the triplet (heroine) mother Valerie Cormack, I asked her what was the hardest part of caring for her babies. I expected a long diatribe about visiting special care units or sleeplessness, but instead she answered: 'Shopping. There is nothing worse than buying three of the same thing, and then realizing that it was a mistake.' And this comes from the woman who gave birth to all three of her babies naturally in hospital.

So, let's get serious about shopping for a moment. After all, you have worked hard for your money, and you don't want to blow it on something you have no hope of returning to the shop after the babies are born. There is a lot of necessary stuff to buy in preparation for twins – pregnancy clothes, cots and nursery furniture, buggies and bathtime accessories – so there is no escape. You might as well enjoy the experience by starting early and acquiring the catalogues and getting the boring but important stuff out of the way now. Then you will have hours to coo over cashmere booties as the pregnancy wears on, knowing that a telephone call to one of your hundreds of catalogue people will solve any last-minute necessities. Sorted.

Maternity wear for big mothers

The best rule is to avoid the twilight world of non-fashion that is maternity wear until you can no longer go a day without those comfy jersey gussets for the stomach. Before that moment you can make do with the latest fantastic invention from Australia, the Bellybelt, an ingenious device that fits over your normal trousers and allows you to keep within the bounds of normal fashion for a few weeks longer. It sells for £12.95 and the box comes with three sizes of elastic and three different materials – white, black or denim (see www.grobag.com).

However, when the Bellybelt and the size 18s and 20s from your favourite shops no longer fit, you have to give up and call in the brochures. Once you have, and you are wearing your first pair of maternity jeans, you will heave a huge sigh of relief. They will feel so comfortable. You can't believe why you didn't succumb to big pants or maternity tights earlier. Don't worry – your partner will thank you for holding out this long. There is nothing in this world less sexy than a drop-down bra.

Sadly for twin mothers, the day of maternity-wear reckoning will be reached far earlier than for those carrying singletons. But you can at least comfort yourself in the knowledge that you will get far more wear out of them. Also, lest you forget, you will be wearing those same maternity trousers for a good few weeks (or months in my case) after you have had the babies. The sight of a twin mother's stomach after the birth is best kept under wraps. It will be a while before the diamond in your pierced tummy button is back out on display.

When it comes to buying maternity wear, go only for the 'capsule wardrobe'. You remember that 90s' fashion phase that urged everyone to go out and buy dark-coloured tailored basics to wear with T-shirts for power breakfasts and board meetings? Well, it may have dropped off the agenda for London Fashion Week, but it is still vital to your pregnant sense of wellbeing. There is nothing worse than waking every morning and having a clothes tantrum because you can't face your multicoloured 'fun' top. You need to invest in some dark-coloured basics, even if the only power breakfast on the horizon is with your pussycat.

The capsule wardrobe

For your capsule wardrobe, the 'maternity' basics are:

- Big pants (I suppose thongs are doable under the bump, but all that rubbing is soon going to make you head towards Bridget Jones's favourite drawer)
- Maternity tights (other tights just don't work)
- Maternity drop-down bra (this is for breastfeeding later, but as your boobs will have already gone up a cup size or two, you may as well buy early rather than buy twice)
- Maternity jeans (see below)

- Maternity stretch trousers (black, don't be tempted by any fawn or 'fun' light colours as they will remain stubbornly in the wardrobe)
- Some tops (don't have to be cut in the maternity bias but may show the unattractive jersey stomach gusset if not)
- Two dresses (optional, but dresses are just so much more comfortable by the end, when even the forgiving gusset has a piece of elastic pressing down on your stomach). Dresses, particularly if they are long with long sleeves, need minimum extra layers, which you don't have in your wardrobe anyway. Plus, with dresses, you can sometimes get away with non-maternity stuff. I wore two Ghost non-maternity dresses right up until my 40th week with the twins, so anything is possible.

The joy of mail order

Whether you live in the city or the country, by the time you have become so pregnant that you don't feel like moving, or later on a housebound mother, you are ready to discover the joy of mail order. It is part necessity and part fantasy (impossibly clean babies, no hint of baby sick anywhere, being pushed along by beautiful blonde teenage model mothers, no sign of bags under the eyes). Once you have rung for your first catalogue, you will become an addict. It is a perfectly normal symptom of shopping deprivation brought about by being too large to undress in tiny cubicles. Fortunately for you, your addiction will be fed forever more by new catalogues from different baby-related manufacturers arriving on your doorstep unasked for. You may tut about the paper wastage, but before long you will be hooked, flicking through the pages to see the latest baby gizmos.

The upside to mail-order shopping is that you can do it when you are pinned to the bed breastfeeding two babies, and you can shop online when the children are asleep. The downside is that once the babies are born, you are unlikely ever to find an envelope and Sellotape to return anything that didn't fit. My twins are still waiting to grow into their cute Breton tops, bought by mistake at size six years instead of six months.

The best maternity-wear and baby shops

Blooming Marvellous
(0870 751 8944: www.bloomingmarvellous.co.uk)

Blooming awful name but it boasts the 'UK's largest range of maternity wear' and has some good classic items for late pregnancy, such as large linen shirts that can also be worn afterwards. It is a one-stop shop for your pregnancy capsule wardrobe with a growing newborn section. Just steer away from Womb Song Kit (£49.99). Your babies will never thank you, and that money would be better spent at the Gucci of pregnancy wear – Formes.

Formes
(0208 689 1133: www.formes.com)

Formes is *the* French maternity-wear company where all pregnant mothers would shop if they were rich celebrities. That doesn't mean you cannot treat yourself to one item there. And if you do buy only one thing, make it a pair of jeans. A pair bought by a friend for £75 is on its fourth pregnant mother, and they still look great. Women who work in the City should only buy maternity wear from Formes, because they can.

Jojo Maman Bébé
(0870 241 0560: www.Jojomamanbebe.co.uk)

Also French, and a little more classy than bloomingterrible-name. Its website is well-organized and easy to buy from. Its denim jeans are cheaper than its French rival at around £32.99.

Brora
(0207 736 9944: www.brora.co.uk)

This company makes exquisite cashmere baby clothes: cardigans (£45), trousers (£45) as well as hand-knitted baby bonnets (£23), baby booties (£19) and baby mittens (£15). One friend who was given a gift box of trousers and cardy loved the feel of her cashmere baby so much that every night for three months she would wash out the top and bottoms and hang them on a radiator for the next day. Some may be horrified at the thought of spending so much on baby clothes, so this is one to be given as a gift, if anybody's asking. Yasmin Le Bon, who discovered Brora for her children, never hands on the clothes but recycles them into cushions. If it's good enough for Yasmin…

Beaming baby
(0800 034 5672: www.beamingbaby.com)

This is a totally organic website offering mainly toiletries for babies – natural bathcare, talcum powder and kits for mothers. It also sells some unusual hand-finished clothes for babies made from organic cotton – its long-sleeved 'bodies', sleepsuits and babygros are an environmentally-friendly alternative to the bigger stores.

Mothercare
(0845 330 4030: www.mothercare.com)

Unless you are reading this after a major relaunch, Mothercare seems to me to have gone off the boil in recent years with some frumpy maternity offerings and often poorly-stocked shops. Shame when you consider that it's the name everyone gropes for when they need anything baby-wise. One pregnant friend became so exasperated with not being able to find a shop assistant recently that she stood in the middle of the store and announced 'I am here to spend hundreds of pounds with you, please can anyone help me?' She spent £800 at the store and had to return to the shop when the goods were delivered because they still had their security tags on.

When I contacted Mothercare about these general issues of stock and customer service, they replied:

'We acknowledge that our performance in these areas has not lived up to the expectations of our customers. We have a new and revitalized senior management team in place that is concentrating its efforts on returning Mothercare to its position of pre-eminence as the number one retailer for parents.'

Watch this space.

Not Mail-order but Worth the Schlep

H&M Hennes – Mama Range
(www.hm.co.uk)

The Hennes maternity line knocks spots off the catalogue stuff price-wise. Pick up basic long-sleeved T-shirts and stretchy trousers for a few quid. It is also much trendier. Think Natalie from All Saints rather than Cherie from Number 10. However, as we go to press, the website only offers a store locator rather than online ordering, so you will need to plan a trip.

Little stuff for tiny babies

You'll be amazed at how little stuff you need to begin with, particularly if you are breastfeeding. Don't be seduced by the magazines. Buy as you go along and second-hand from twins club newsletters, if you can. There are some things that only the catalogues sell, however. I've listed below the best buys that do the rounds through our local club's quarterly journal.

The swing chair

This is a battery-powered rocking chair, suitable from birth-ish up until 25lb in weight. The benefit for a twin mother is that you can put one baby in it, rocking happily away on one of two speeds, with annoying jangly music, while changing the other. The downside is that they take up about as much room as a small helicopter in your living room. Brand new, they cost around £89 from catalogues such as Perfectly Happy People (0870 607 0545: wwwthebabycatalogue.com). Second-hand, they sell for around £50.

The V-shaped cushion

This is used for breastfeeding and propping up one little baby while you feed the other. One twin mother even uses hers to stop her two-year-old falling out of bed (one arm is a pillow, the other a buffer). She also found a rare V-shaped cushion with Velcro straps, allowing her to walk around the house with it strapped on like an ocean-going liner. Poor husband. The V-shaped cushion always comes out as a best buy for twin mothers because it allows you to breastfeed both babies at the same time (the double football hold), no-handed. Even if you bottle-feed, you can prop up both babies facing each other while you hold the bottles. Oh, what versatility! As well as being on sale at WI meetings for oldies who like to read in bed, it is also found at John Lewis stores and catalogues such as Perfectly Happy People (*see above*).

The baby change station

If you only had one baby, you might get away with not having to invest in a baby change station (the cheapest being a canvas and metal foldaway number costing around £30 in IKEA). However, if you don't invest in one with twins, you would spend triple the cost at the osteopath after 100 nappy changes in the first week alone. If you can possibly afford it, buying one for upstairs and one for downstairs will also see you through the blizzard of nappies in the first few months.

Bath safety seats

Bathing twins in the early days is a two-person job unless you invest in bath seats. I bought two from Cheeky Rascals

(£12.95 mail-order: 01428 682488) and I credit the purchase with helping my twins love water. The seat, which has recently won *Parenting* magazine Best Buy, is made of moulded plastic and props the baby in a semi-upright position. The baby is supported under the arms and legs, which are free to flail about, but cannot slip downwards. Once the twins get used to the water (my little girl used to scream when first immersed for about a week), they can splash around to their hearts' content. In the early days, this means you could down a whole cup of tea. Well worth every penny.

The real nappy issue

You may be wondering at this stage what on earth makes one nappy brand better than another (the answer is whichever has a freebie of some wipes attached to them). Or you may be thinking that you'd like to do your bit for the environment and use real nappies. Whatever your view, you are entering a fiercely competitive world where the big brands like Pampers will be vying for your loyalty along with the little local nappy laundering services. Whatever you decide, remember that you will only have time to research the options before the babies are born. After that, it will be whatever the local store has in stock.

Biodegradable disposables

There is only one brand of disposable nappy that is biodegradable, and it is called Nature's Boy and Girl. They are unisex (useful for boy/girl twins) and sold in all the big supermarkets, but sadly not in smaller chemists. Invented by a Swedish woman called Marlien Sandberg, the nappy is 70 per cent biodegradable, and a new prototype – 100 per cent biodegradable – may even be in production at the time of reading. For those too overstretched to want to wash or fold nappies, these are a good compromise. You are doing your bit for the environment, and can sleep at night knowing that of the 800,000 tonnes of nappy waste collected every year in UK landfill sites, at least your babies' contributions will be rotting down. The shocking alternative is the knowledge that the very first disposable nappy ever made has yet to biode-grade.

Real nappy laundering agencies

For the first nine months of the twins' lives, I opted for a nappy laundering service, which delivered 100 nappies for the babies every week and took away the soiled ones. As well as the laundering service, I also rented 12 plastic pants to put the nappies in, and they worked well with no problem of rashes or leakages. I even quite liked the chore of folding these white cotton nappy liners; it gave me a whiff of what it would be like to be a real earth mother. However, my main problem was the smell. The buckets that had to wait for a week for collection began to pong so badly that they eventually had to be put at the end of the garden near the compost. And if I forgot to put the nappy bucket out for collection, then the garden became a horsebox. The total cost was around £8 per week per baby, around the same cost as disposables. For your nearest nappy collection and delivery scheme, call The National Association of Nappy Services (0121 693 4949).

Real nappies to buy

In the year 2000, there were 10 companies selling cloth nappies; today there are about 22. Some mothers go for buying and using the cloth nappies because it works out cheaper in the long run. Friends of the Earth estimate that cloth nappies cost an average of £400 per baby over a two-year period before a baby is potty-trained, including the cost of washing powder, electricity, water and wear and tear (estimated at £40). Disposables cost £1,200 per baby for a two-year period – no small figure when doubled.

These days 'real nappy systems', as they are grandly called, have come a long way from the terry-towelling-and-safety-pin days of our mothers. Lively animal prints make them a little more fun to hang out on the washing line, and the Velcro or popper fastenings are a doddle to do. Catalogues such as PHP (0870 6070545), Cheeky Rascals (01428 682488) and Little Green Earthlets (01825 873301: www.earthlets.co.uk) carry a range, but for background information contact The Real Nappy Association (0208 299 4519).

One of the biggest manufacturers, Kooshies (0870 607 0545), often provides a sample pack for interested mothers. Those wishing to turn their interest into a lifetime of placard-waving on behalf of the environment can also get the low-down on the impact of disposables on the planet from the Women's Environment Network (0207 481 9004).

The wonderful world of double buggies

If you thought buying a car was difficult (am I a hatchback sort of person or a sports car kind of girl?), then the double buggy showroom will send you rushing to the nearest shrink. Double buggies seem to cost about as much as a car, need at least an O-level in engineering to put up and down, and generate very little interest in the male species. If you do have a man with strong opinions about what you should buy, think twice about doing as you're told against your better judgment. Exactly how much pushing up and down the pavements and hills will he be doing with it? A Saturday stroll is quite different from a slog back from Sainsbury's with the weekly shop.

One reason why the world of double buggies is so complicated is because manufacturers are always bringing out new pushchairs with fabrics and features that instantly make last year's model look like stale buns. We have a video in our twins club library called *Coping with Twins* (don't bother, it's from the 1970s), which shows a mother trying to ram a new double buggy through her front door. Under the helpful banner of 'make sure your double buggy can fit through an average door', this poor woman is trying to negotiate a vehicle the size of two shopping trolleys up the front step. Meanwhile, her twins are lying down *on their fronts* in the buggy, with their heads bobbing up and down like nodding dogs.

In a recent local twins club survey, two mothers groaned about how the Mothercare Urban Detour model was 82 cms wide and didn't fit through their front doors. The thought of unloading your twins in the rain, and taking the shopping off the back of the buggy while finding the keys in the bottom of your handbag is no small consideration, so don't rely on manufacturers to build to standard-width doors. At the risk of making the book instantly out of date, because by the time you read this some company will have just brought out a model with a pump-action pellet gun to zap other buggies out of the way, let me offer the results of our own twins club survey a little later on (*see pages 56–7*). In defence of being yesterday's news, note that manufacturers' 'new ranges' tend to offer cosmetic changes, such as different fabrics, rather than radical design improvements.

The first three months

The pram you need for the first three months of your babies' life is quite different from the one you need for the next two years. Some manufacturers do try and get round this by getting their sitting-up versions to lie flat, but it can often look like a compromise. Although you will be focused on the babies as tiny little beans that need protecting, if you are buying new, do look ahead to the moment they can sit up – around six months.

Many twin mothers get round the problem by renting a pram (not particularly cheap) or borrowing for those first three months, and then buying the three-wheeler of their choice when the babies are six months old. For the first three months you will want your babies to be lying together, replicating the experience in the womb, so that they sleep more soundly comforted by each other's presence. For that reason, old-fashioned prams – or even single prams for a month or two – often do the trick of keeping them tucked up cosily as twins. Once the babies are sitting up, a whole new world of buggies open up to you, and these buggies can then last the next two years.

Buy second-hand

One of the advantages of living on our crowded, small island is that neighbours and friends are always keen to offload equipment to make space in their shed. This is particularly true when your news of expecting twins reaches the outside world. Offers will come from the most unexpected sources – I was offered a front-and-back buggy in shocking purple and green from my sister-in-law's former au pair's current employer (see what I mean about 'unexpected'). Then a friend turned up with a side-by-side Maclaren umbrella double buggy. As it turned out, both were useful. The front and back one lasted no more than six months because it became too heavy to lift up and down pavements. The second side-by-side number is still brought out for emergencies (and I was interested to see in our twins club survey that 45 per cent of mothers had a Maclaren as a second buggy).

Remember, most double buggies are not designed for twins but for mothers who have two children in rapid succession, and are weighted in favour of a 'light' child and a 'heavy' child. The very best place to buy a second-hand buggy is from your local twins club newsletter. That way you can visit the mother who owned it and get the whole low-down on how to put it up and down and whether it works through thick mud in the fog.

Buy cheap, buy twice

When I bought my twin buggy new off an American site on the internet, and had it couriered over to an address where we were holidaying in the States, I thought I was the cleverest mother on the block. It only cost me $100, it was front-and-back with a twist (the babies could face each other) and it even had a special place to put my coffee cup from Starbucks. I was in heaven. Although only for 10 weeks. After 10 weeks, constant abuse from the twins bouncing up and down and my four-year-old insisting that he had a ride meant the chassis broke and my dreams were dashed. Because I bought it in America and on the internet, I had no comeback. It still sits in my shed as a horrible reminder of that 'buy cheap, buy twice' motto.

If you do buy a double buggy that doesn't come from a recognized manufacturer, you may be entering the world of cheap, dodgy metal frames and wheels that can't be replaced. Just remember that it should last for at least two years, until your twins refuse point blank to be strapped into it. Before buying, check out all the brands and prices through the internet to get the cheapest price for the model. After three second-hand buggies and one new, we have finally invested in a nearly-new, smart three-wheeler Land Rover buggy for £200 (it costs £400 new). This is hopefully our last purchase. Had we bought it brand new at the beginning, it would have come out cheaper in total than all the other second-hand models and American trash that fell by the wayside. If you make only one new purchase, make it a double buggy.

Front and back versus side by side

This debate rages at every twin-club coffee morning in the country. A distillation of the advantages and disadvantages goes something like this:

- **Front-and-back** buggies are heavier and longer, so they hurt backs and don't fit into most small cars.
- They are, however, easier to get in and out of shops and always have one handle with which to push them (so you can drink your coffee or gabble on the mobile when out and about).
- F'n'B buggies feel a bit more private – the back compartment at least – so babies can sleep a little more undisturbed.
- As the babies get slightly older, front and back buggies have the added advantage of separating your twins so that they don't pull each other's hair, thus avoiding the heart-stopping yelps that accompany my school run in the side-by-side number every day.
- **Side-by-side buggies** tend to be lighter if they are the umbrella-type, so they fold away more neatly, are useful for travelling abroad, and can be stacked in a hallway or hung up without bringing the wall down.
- They are easier to get up and down kerbs than front-and-backs because the weight is more evenly distributed (three wheelers are even easier than side-by-sides).
- They are harder to get in and out of shops because of their size.
- The umbrella-sort have three handles instead of one, so multi-tasking one-handed is out.

Two up front and one on the back

It's all very well making sure your twins are comfortably seated in their double buggy, but what happens when you also have an older child who's not ready to be kicked out onto the street yet? The answer is the Buggy- or Kiddie-board, a skateboard-like contraption that fits onto the rear axle of your pushchair and is the true definition of a free ride. Up until now, however, the choice of buggies that allow you to attach the board has been severely limited. Not only that, the moment you attach the Buggy-board, your manufacturer's guarantee is invalidated – so if a wheel falls off on day two, you're on your own and very probably in the gutter. Until now that is, following the news that manufacturer Mountain Buggy, that produces three-wheelers, has redesigned these buggies to allow the addition of a Kiddie-board – guarantee intact. No doubt other manufacturers will follow suit shortly.

To buy the new Buggy-board with enough adaptability to fit most double buggies (£44.95) or the double buggy adaptors (£6.95) for second-hand buggy-boards, call the mail-order company Cheeky Rascals (01428 682488; www.cheekyrascals.co.uk). The company also operates a buggy-board hotline for clueless parents who can't wield a spanner.

The survey

According to our local survey of 50 mothers, which is not scientific and only reflects our views, the prams and pushchairs used are, in order of popularity:

○ **Maclaren** – this is the most popular 'second' buggy because it is versatile for shopping and travel and folds down to a very neat, small size. However, some moan that it becomes heavy to push when the twins get bigger and may not last the full two-year course with vigorous use – especially if a buggy board is attached. After only one year, twin mother Susie Boone took hers in for a service locally and was told that the wheels needed replacing because they had worn down. Maclaren's answer:

'By definition a double buggy will be subjected to a harder life than a single, as it is carrying both a larger combined weight and being used by effectively twice as many children. It is therefore even more important to take preventative measures to guarantee the longevity of your buggies.'

They are covered by a six-month warranty and a service can be arranged by calling Maclaren customer services on 01327 841320.

○ **Bébé Confort** – one of the few models that adapts from a totally flat pram to a seated buggy, so is suitable from birth to two years old. It is genuinely designed for twins, is narrower than the average side by side so fits through most doors, but looks rather old fashioned. The handle on ours dropped to knee level as the twins approached two and became heavier and heavier.

○ **Silver Cross** – every granny's favourite. A bit heavy and old fashioned, but good for walking cross country.

○ **Graco** – gets heavy as the twins get older.

- **Mamas and Papas** – similar to the Maclaren but bigger wheels means easier pushing and steering.
- **Emmaljunga** – big wheels make it sturdy for walking.
- **Mothercare Atlanta** – some had problems with the frame and Mothercare no longer stock this model.

Three-wheeler versus four-wheeler

Ever since Tom Cruise was caught in *Hello!* magazine years ago, roller-blading around Hyde Park with headphones on and pushing his progeny in a three-wheeler buggy, the parks have never looked the same again. Three-wheelers, once the domain of celebrities and rich kids because of their price, are now produced by hundreds of different manufacturers all keen to dazzle you with the latest big wheel.

Our own 2003 twins club survey of 50 mothers proved that three-wheelers were now the most popular type of buggy among twin mothers. In the questionnaire, most mothers stated that their biggest advantage is how easy they are to push – no small point if you have hills or muddy tracks to climb. The downside is that they are long, and some will only fit into a people carrier or estate car.

Most three-wheeler double buggies sit side by side, with one notable exception. The Kiwi Explorer, an import from New Zealand now available over here at a price, carries the second child underneath the first in a sort of kangaroo pouch. It is not suitable from birth, but the mother using it at our twins club, Megan, who has identical twin boys, is still piling them into it aged two-and-a-half. She claims that by hiding one underneath the other she saves herself hours of being stopped by passers-by cooing at the boys' shock of blond hair. When you hear of a triplet mother once being stopped 57 times as she made her way across Brent Cross Shopping Centre in north London, you can see that this is some hidden advantage.

The three-wheelers in order of popularity are:

Mountain Buggy: Twin Terrain/Urban – expensive, but well worth it as the twins get heavier. It is light, easy to push but takes up a lot of boot space. The Terrain has a fixed front wheel; the urban a swivel front wheel.

Mothercare (Urban Detour/Alpine) – great mobility but does not fit through some doorways.

Pegasus All Terrain

Nipper Double – All Terrain buggy – comfy for sleeping and relatively cheap for what it is.

Inset Ultra (USA import)

Alurax

Land Rover – buy British. I bought this and found two niggles. The sheath-like unlocking mechanism needed repairing and the shopping tray underneath has to be un-Velcroed before putting down.

Buggies and travel

If you do intend to travel around with your twins and can't afford a second Maclaren umbrella-style double buggy, invest in a couple of cheap single umbrella-style numbers from Argos. The cheapest are around £15 and are often better suited for foreign pavements and doorways – as long as you have an extra pair of hands to push them. At the airport on the way to Spain, I had to call upon the assistance of my four-year-old to push one of the twins to check-in. For the record, it is physically impossible to push a luggage trolley and a buggy.

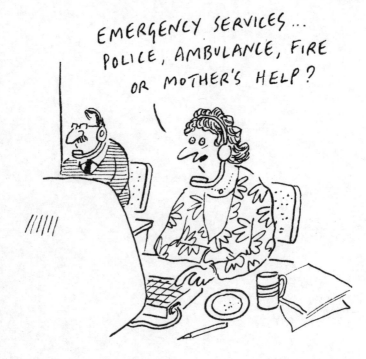

Help! I Need Help!

Because Western 'civilization' is the only culture in the world that expects new mothers to cope on their own, all of us doing identical jobs in our identical houses with our identical time-saving machines and with no-one to talk to, I am going to say the unsayable. Under no circumstances should you plan to take your twins back home and cope on your own. In fact, I am so convinced that our rotten-to-mothers culture is wrong that I forbid you to skip over this chapter. A few months down the line, when you are limbering up for the SuperMum of the Year awards (note – they don't exist), you can show off your double nappy change in under two minutes to the cat. But certainly in the first few months, you must assume you will need help.

One great thing about twins is that, unlike the rest of the poor mothers of singletons, you can play the Mother-of-Twins card on the help front. This card, which can be employed at any tricky moment in the first three years, is the 'Oh yes, they are such hard work . . . I couldn't do it without my wonderful nanny/childminder/au pair/mother/husband.' No-one ever argues, because no-one can claim to know what it is like. And the more you ham it up to be double trouble, the more sympathy, rather than envy, you attract. Occasionally, when you have left your sitting room looking like a skip and are out in the world to escape your domestic chaos, a kind word from another mother makes all the difference. 'I don't know how you manage with two' always gives extra va-va-voom to my supermarket trolley.

If you are a mother expecting triplets, you need no excuse. You only need to know that someone totted up the number of hours needed to feed, change and look after three babies in the early days and it came to 28 hours in a 24-hour day. It's like that Monty Python sketch of the men sitting around comparing whose youth was harder: 'We used to have to get up before we went to bed...'

Because it is traditional to assume that 'help' is a little luxury for ladies who lunch, and not a god-given right to all new mothers, I will wade in first and foremost with the most expensive and qualified sort of help that you deserve, before looking at the most likely sort of help you will get – grannies, relatives and husbands. You will have to forgive me for putting husbands last. I have visited many twin mothers with baby-loving and nappy-changing Dads, but I don't have one at home. Unreconstructed Yorkshiremen who beg to sleep 'in a broom cupboard if it doesn't have a baby in there' are unlikely to be seen around town wearing a papoose. The benefit for you the reader is that, as a result, I have had every sort of help through my front door. I am a veteran of the nanny/granny power struggle and the au pair's boyfriend problems.

Sort out your help early

The first thing to learn about help, which is why this chapter is sneaked in before the birth, is that you have to sort it out way before you go into labour. Not because you will be too busy to sort it out afterwards, but because you may not like the person. This is no small matter. All of us think we are pretty good judges of character, but until you have actually had the nanny clomping around your sitting room in high heels, or shrinking the hand-knitted jumpers in the tumble dryer, you never know. One twin mother knew the moment her maternity nurse appeared down the stairs in a starched white uniform, likening her to Nurse Ratchet from *One Flew Over the Cuckoo's Nest*.

A couple of afternoons of getting the new nanny over to sort out the nursery or help you choose a pram will give you some inkling of how you rub along together. Also, even if you have met her, decided against her, and then need to call her back in desperation after the birth – you have at least done some sort of vetting.

Another reason for starting early is because you may have to search a little longer to find someone happy to look after twins. There is always the danger that those who see nannying as a job rather than a joy may be put off by twins, and think 'two for the price of one'. For triplets, it's worse – two mothers of triplets put identical adverts in *The Lady* for a nanny. One admitted to expecting triplets, the other didn't. The first received over 100 enquiries; the other, just four. But the four candidates were all keen, and the keenest is spooning puréed carrot into a baby's mouth right now.

Leaving yourself a little extra time to find the right person will put your mind at ease. You don't want anyone who isn't delighted at the prospect of looking after your precious bundles. And, believe it or not, because twin mothers are seen as generally relaxed about handing over a baby for cuddling and winding, there are plenty of candidates out there.

Those of us also lucky enough to have a devoted granny in the wings, waiting for her moment to have both babies on her knees and the camera flashes popping, are blessed indeed. All grannies, including mother-in-law grannies, are far preferable to a moping au pair at the top of the house. And grannies are great for the baby times. When you have two vandals as toddlers on your hands, granny and grandpa might take up golf suddenly. But in the baby months, just try keeping them away.

What if I want to muddle through on my own?

If these are your first children, and you really would rather rub along happy but messy, sleeping when the twins do, eating takeaways and supermarket meals, with no-one to think about but your babies, and no-one to judge you as the dishes pile up, then there is no reason why you can't cope on your own. Could I just make a tiny proviso and suggest a cleaner for that very initial period after the birth when you still deserve a little spoiling? If you already have one, then ask her in advance if she might pop in three times a week, rather than once. If you don't, see whether you might find one that has also been a mother, so that you can ask her advice about the colour of twin one's poo (you will get there, I promise) as well as the type of washing powder you should be using.

I have a dear friend from school who is a talented painter. She hadn't picked up a paintbrush for 10 years, since her first daughter was born. The day she got a cleaner for the first time, a few weeks before her second son was due, she painted four wonderfully colourful charcoal drawings that now adorn her kitchen walls. Just having the support of another woman or girlfriend during the transition to new motherhood is immensely reassuring. Who knows what we are capable of with a little help. Go on – get a cleaner for those last few weeks of pregnancy and first weeks of motherhood. In the words of Jennifer Aniston, 'Why? Because you're worth it.'

Help for the first few months

I felt quite strongly that I needed someone with a bit of experience for twins, rather than a rookie staring at me as I squinted to read the instructions for the double buggy. I preferably wanted someone who had had children herself, and so would find handling a baby quite natural, and could say the right thing when I asked for the third time: 'Do you think he's crying because he's still hungry?' I didn't want to look like I was permanently playing charades, explaining everything in semaphore language to an au pair that didn't speak English.

After those initial three months, when life gets a little easier, I knew I could always look for a different sort of help if I needed it. To start with, holed away in our Victorian house, I wanted a live-out mother's help, so we weren't moving from a two-adult, one-child family to a crowded three-adult, three-children set up. I felt that once we had weathered the transition we could then adopt the 'come one, come all' approach to communal living and get a young au pair who could be 'trained up' in the ways of the household. If she had arrived before the twins were nine months old, the only training she would have got would be in the theory of Brownian motion – lots of people bumping into each other in corridors at all hours of the day and night.

Maternity nurses

No maternity nurse gets out of bed for less than £600 per week, and some of the most highly recommended charge up to £1,000 per week in central London. Wow, you think. You and your husband are in the wrong job. What's more, one mother of twins who tried to book someone recommended by a friend was told that the maternity nurse was booked up for 12 months ahead (a couple who were just about to begin trying for a baby had booked her 'just in case'). For your foresight and money in booking a maternity nurse, you get someone on duty for 24 hours a day, six days a week to care for mother and baby. Washing up and cooking the meals is not on the agenda, although most do spirit themselves away tactfully when the husband arrives home from work.

Many people who run nanny agencies think that maternity nurses have had their day and are being replaced more and more by 'doulas' (*see below*). Traditionally, maternity nurses would come and stay for six weeks once the husband had gone back to work. You have to book them around your due date, so there is always a danger of paying them to twiddle their thumbs if you are overdue, or failing to have them around if you are early. One first-time mother who wrote about her maternity nurse in our twin club newsletter, and had paid £2,000 for four weeks, said that she would really rather have had a bit of extra help during the day with shopping, washing and cooking instead of looking after the babies.

She suggests asking yourself the following questions before booking one:

- How easily and comfortably can you accommodate another adult in your home?
- Will the lack of privacy be a problem for you and your partner?
- Do you intend to breastfeed at night and therefore have to get up anyway (maternity nurses are traditionally the only source of help for the nights as well as the days)?
- Do you have a friend or relative who would be happy to help out instead?

She wrote 'Perhaps if I had spoken to a first-time mum with twins, rather than just mothers of singletons, I would not have been scared silly and started off by believing that I couldn't cope. I might have saved myself a few thousand pounds in the process.'

Most of all, unless they are recommended by a friend, you need to check out their references thoroughly, quizzing previous employers on the phone. My dear sister-in-law sent her young maternity nurse packing after a week when she found her high heels in the country and refusal to sleep in the same room as the baby too much to bear. Perhaps if she had grilled the other mothers who had had her, or, even better, met her first, the sudden departure might have been avoided.

If the cost of a maternity nurse hasn't sent you straight down to the au pair section, then it is time to say a few things in their defence. The friends who have hired them and the twin mother in our survey who could not praise her maternity nurse too highly, have had an experienced hand to talk through every detail and support them 24 hours a day as they attempt to breastfeed. Most maternity nurses believe in establishing routines (those that can't afford nurses can learn their tricks through the *Contented Little Baby Book, see Chapter 13*) and, by the time they leave, they will have miraculously turned your two squalling infants into, well, contented little babies. And if it all works out, the only person crying on her departure will be you, the mother. Maternity nurses are found through local nanny agencies.

Live-in/live-out nannies

Oh, for Mary Poppins. All laughter and sensible routines and fun days out for the children. Where is she? Why doesn't she exist? And do you think she'd take a job in Sunderland? I actually blubbed when watching *Mary Poppins* while pregnant with the twins because I knew I could never have her. Today's nannies are more likely to be young girls from Australia or New Zealand who are spending a little time in the old country before heading off on their travels around the world.

The main thing that distinguishes a nanny from other forms of help is that they speak perfect English. These days, many nanny agencies will offer the services of people who may not have NNEB qualifications but are mothers returning to work after raising their own children, or au pairs who have been in the country for a couple of years and speak good English.

The other distinction between a nanny and other forms of help is that they should be able to be left in 'sole charge' (you may as well start learning the lingo now) of babies while you go out – for 10 minutes or for a whole day at work. If they have no qualifications, you should insist on two references and speak to their former employers on the telephone. Written references are for the Mary Poppins era. You want to ask the mother who employed her why she left her employment, how loving and warm she was, and what the mother would say her weaknesses – as well as her strengths – are.

The other big distinction between nannies and the rest is their cost. Since the government recently brought in the hated 'nanny tax', the cost of nannies to be paid out of your taxed disposable income is high. And there are few tax breaks. Unless you work from home as a self-employed business and could claim that you run a crèche from your premises, there are no avoidance schemes. You have to pay their tax, holiday pay and national insurance contributions as employer and employee. So, for example, one triplet mother I know pays her nanny £200 per week net. On top of that she has to pay £30.10 per week tax and £34.33 for employer's and employee's national insurance contributions – a total of £264.43. Nannies are one of the few workers that always discuss their payment in 'net' or take-home terms rather than gross income.

A few years ago, you might have paid £50 less for a live-in nanny for providing room and board, but these days it is assumed you are paying for their expertise, and there is little difference in the salary. Nannies are found through agencies in your Yellow Pages, or through advertisements in *The Lady*.

Nanny share

If you are going back to work part-time, or want a qualified person to help you with the babies only a few days a week, it is possible to go for a nanny share. Agencies can usually help find you a part-time nanny, although a lot of mothers organize it on their own, advertising in health clubs, post offices and second-hand baby equipment shops. The advantages of knowing the other half of your nanny share is obvious. If you are not both going out to work and are therefore flexible in your days, a little bit of boxing and coxing can be arranged between you if you want to try a new aquababies class on a Friday. Naturally, the same rules for tax and national insurance apply, but these are shared by both parties.

Nanny trainees

Colleges that are training girls to be nursery nurses or nannies love mothers of twins. Twin mothers are usually generous (grateful) in allowing others to handle a baby under their watchful eye because they are busy with the other. For this reason, many nursery colleges target twin mothers through advertisements in the local twins club newsletters for work placements for their students. To get a BTEC in child-care or an NVQ level 2 or 3, and therefore on the books of a nanny agency, a young girl needs to have had experience with a baby.

The placements amount to two or three mornings and afternoons a week over a minimum two-week period, usually just after the birth. The placements are free, although some mothers offer to pay travel expenses for the student, and again it is good to call well ahead to be put on the college register. To find out about nursery trainee placements call your local further education college.

Doulas

Doulas (pronounced doo-la) are an American invention that appeared on the scene a few years ago. Up until then we had our own homely sounding 'mother's help', traditionally a girl of 16 who had left home and was looking for work before deciding on a career. Mother's helps are older or 'more mature' these days because nobody leaves school at 16 anymore, and if they do decide to specialize in childcare, they come out with BTECs or NVQs looking for nannying jobs.

The beauty of doulas is that they do all sorts of jobs, not just looking after mother and baby, and are just as likely to be cleaning out the gunk in the dishwasher as giving the twins a bottle. Doulas even come with a qualification from a 'doula course' these days, although technically speaking it is not a nationally-recognized one.

Nevertheless, at £8 to £10 per hour, and an assumption that they come before and after the birth (good for vetting) and stay for as long as you want, they are becoming a popular choice. Local nanny agencies now offer doulas on their books or you could put an advertisement in your local free newspaper or newsagent's window for a mother's help looking for extra work during school hours.

Au pairs

Au pairs are a total lottery. If you are lucky enough to strike gold the first time, you will think you have cracked the help thing for the rest of your life, and that au pairs are the best (and cheapest) invention known to woman. However, should you house a girl who is sorry to be a long way from home, with no urge to make friends, you will find yourself caught between resentment for thinking up meals for you both to eat and exhaustion at trying to cheer her up.

Our first au pair, a very depressed Emmy from Denmark, got engaged moments before coming over, and spent the whole time rolling cigarettes and looking wistfully out of the window. It was only when my husband complained that he was fed up with looking after the baby while I drove the au pair to keep fit classes and the hairdressers to put a smile on her face that I realized something was wrong. The lesson I learnt early on was that if they are going to stay, then no amount of cooking shepherd's pie or listening to Kiss FM to please them has any effect. They will stay because they like being away from their family, making friends and going out. To keep them in and to improve their English, it is always worth sticking a telly in their room.

Without going into racial stereotypes over au pairs, I will just put in a quick plug for the new breed of super au pair – the Eastern European girls. Unspoilt, warm and loving to children, they are delighted with their two-year visas to be in the country and hardworking to boot. Au pairs traditionally work five hours a day for £50 per week doing 'light housework' (more jargon) and childcare, although you can arrange for them to do extra hours as an 'au pair plus'. We pay our Slovakian au pair Andrea an extra £5 per hour for extra work on top of her five hours a day. When you consider that the average teacher in Slovakia earns only £80 per month, you can see why young girls are keen to be here. Au pairs are expected to do a couple of nights' baby-sitting into the bargain, and as you begin to feel your old mojo returning, they can be a godsend for letting you escape to the cinema for a snooze with your husband.

Finally, au pairs are protected by the Home Office. They are not technically seen as employees but as members of the family, with their own bedroom and living-in expenses such as food paid for on top of their 'pocket money'. Sleep-deprived husbands do not always welcome their evening meals taken up with polite questions about their progress in English classes, so it is worth establishing from the outset whether they are expected for supper.

Nurseries

Nurseries are a good, but expensive, option for twins if you are thinking of returning to work. Many nurseries take very small babies from soon after birth, and some mothers feel reassured that they have more than one member of staff sharing the round-the-clock process of caring for their children. Some nurseries are like public schools, however, and expect you to already have little Timmy's name down for them before your 12-week scan. One mother I know, Sarah, slammed down the phone when a nursery replied haughtily that there was no space for her little girl for another year. 'I thought you were a nursery, not Eton,' she shouted as she hung up.

The best way to judge a nursery is to ignore its glossy brochure and ask to look around the place yourself. Staff turnover is normally a good indicator of the happiness of the place, or you may decide on the spot that a nursery is too open and public. One mother of twins vowed never to let her daughter be cared for by a nursery when she popped in to visit her one lunchtime during work and found her strapped into a chair, covered in apple sauce. She felt so distressed at the sight of her normally fastidious and clean baby shackled and covered in mess that she left her job soon after.

Another advantage of nurseries, apart from the impossibly beautiful artwork that comes home daily with your four-month-old, is that they offer cast-iron reliability – no small bonus if you are holding down a job where that matters. Nurseries never call in sick for the day, leaving you with no choice but to cancel your work. Plus, if you prefer to be in control of your timekeeping, dropping your children off at a nursery, rather than hopping from foot to foot waiting to play relay with the nanny, may suit you better. Do check what time they close, however, as many shut at 6pm, no good for late workers. As one who has never been on time for anything, I have suffered at the hands of my local money-laundering nursery where a stringent fine is charged for late pick-up. On my last day at work, heavily pregnant with the twins, I stopped to telephone the nursery to say I would be 15 minutes late. I was presented with a £70 bill the next day, which, needless to say, I never paid. You have been warned.

The downside of nurseries is their cost – despite the '10 per cent discount' for twins that many offer. A friend Fiona has her twins and three-year-old in nursery while she works part-time for Cadbury Schweppes. She makes £1,500 per month and pays out £1,600 per month in nursery fees. What we will pay to get out of the house these days.

Live-in student help

The lowest form of help, which is unlikely to be suitable for the first year, is live-in student help. Here in Wandsworth, south-west London, and undoubtedly in other parts of the country where foreign students are common, we have local language centres, such as ELT, that require foreign students to live with a local family. ELT runs a scheme where a language student lives in your house and provides 10 hours a week of help with children and light housework plus two evenings baby-sitting. In return you provide a room and food, so no money exchanges hands.

Caroline Watton, a mother of twins and two boys, was concerned this would mean preparing and hosting a meal every evening, but this isn't the case – it is up to you to ensure there is a good supply of food in the house but not to cook for them. Caroline is on her seventh student now, and apart from one homesick Belgian girl, the scheme has worked well.

The godsend in her case is help with bath-times and free baby-sitting with a familiar adult.

Says Caroline: 'So far for me this has been a very different experience compared to the first weeks with a new au pair. It feels less stressful, which is probably down to the following: it's a relief that the girls have not just me but the college to turn to if they run into any problems; there's a ready-made social life through ELT which means I don't have to network for them; and the courses are quite demanding, with a lot of homework, so I don't worry that she is at a loss for things to do. Another key point is that my expectations have been quite low, which is probably the best way to approach this type of help – as long as whoever lives with us is considerate, willing and more of a help than hindrance, then that is enough for me – especially when no money is changing hands. As far as looking after the children is concerned, so long as I feel happy about general attitude and common sense so I can leave the house for a short time and feel secure about evening baby-sitting, then that too is fine.'

Obviously, not all areas of the country will attract foreign students, but this kind of help is worth investigating in university towns as well.

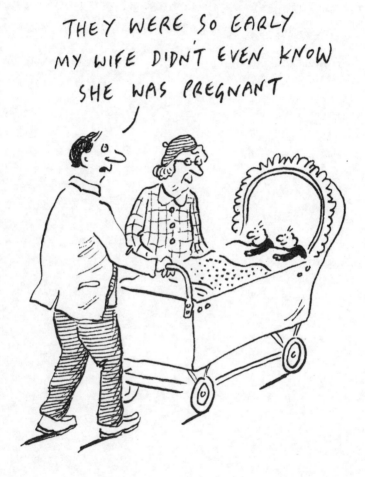

Positive Prem Baby Talk

For all the healthy eating and moderate exercise, for all the au pairs doing the heavy housework, we still have to face facts that half of all twins are born early (before 37 weeks) with a low birth weight ($5^{1}/_{2}$lb/2.5kg or below). That's the bad news. The good news is that if they are born early (or 'prem' or 'preemies' as the pros call them), they will already have matured that much more than single babies born spontaneously at the same age.

Studies have shown that multiple babies have a survival advantage over single babies because of their growth during the second trimester. It is almost as if the body knows that the twins may be born early, and compensates by feeding them up better towards the end. The research that shows this[1] confirms how extra clever twins are, even in utero.

Also, when you are next told the catalogue of complaints that premature babies may suffer from (rather like reading the list of contraindications on the back of a pill packet), remember that the list is drawn up after observing single premature babies (and not extra-clever, extra-mature twins). Most singletons are born prematurely because of poor maternal nutrition, toxaemia and other complications. Twin babies appear early in this world for the simple reason that there is no more room in the womb.

Good figures help

If it is reassuring statistics you need, there are plenty. There is a 98 per cent survival rate for babies born weighing between 2½lb/1kg and 5½lb/2.5kg. Those figures are for all prem babies – no distinction is made to allow for our tougher twin ones.[2] And our local twins club survey showed that only 25 per cent of twins in our area were born before 35 weeks. That means that there were many more twins born that didn't need to spend time in a special care unit than did. So, it is not a given that you will spend extra time in hospital. The average combined weight of twins in our survey, regardless of how the mother had conceived, was 10lb/4.5kg – that's two healthy 5lb/2.2kg babies. And the maximum weight of babies carried by Joanne Pinkness (*see birth stories*) was 15lb/6.8kg! Our bodies really are amazing.

The reasons for wanting to go to term are obvious. Bigger babies mean less time in hospital, and less pressure on you as a new mother to have your babies' weight monitored the whole time. Plus you get to show off to singleton mothers, who only carry one 8lb/3.5kg baby, what an absolute übermama you are.

No blame

I am positive about the prospects of premature babies to thrive because I am the daughter of one. My father was born weighing 2^1/$_2$lb/1kg in 1934, well before the extra technology in today's special care units. He still runs or plays golf every day (so no problem with his lungs, the last organs to mature), and has fathered twins (so no runt of the family there either).

Most likely if the babies do come early, it will be because of factors outside your control (genetics and your size). However, do not assume or let others assume that just because you are carrying twins you will not go to term. My doctor told me that they 'considered term for twins to be 36 weeks', when I went to over 40 weeks. There is nothing wrong with correcting every person and protecting your babies against such harmful assumptions with the simple phrase, 'Well I plan to go to the full 40 weeks.' Gaia Pollini, who went to 40 weeks plus with her twins, practised 'building up a protective shield from negative comments. To anyone who told me that twins come early, I answered "Not mine!".'

For those whose pregnancy demon is that their twins will arrive early, it is worth reading about the great care that Judy Collins received when her two boys, her first children, arrived before she had bought cots or attended the first antenatal class. Judy, like most mothers of premature babies, is a successful breastfeeder and was still feeding her twins at nine months when I came to visit. Great encouragement is given to mothers of premature babies in the early days to feed the babies with breast milk. If the babies are younger than 34 weeks, their sucking reflex has yet to develop, so most preemies are fed by milk expressed with the help of a breast pump, and delivered through a nasal tube. Below is Judy's story.

Judy, 34, found out she was pregnant when she came back from honeymoon with her husband Jim. She had her twin non-identical boys, Thomas and Harry, when 31 weeks pregnant. Thomas weighed 2lb 12oz/1.2kg and Harry 3lb 4oz/1.5kg. The babies were allowed home after 5^1/$_2$ weeks.

I found out I was carrying twins at the 12-week scan. We had to go back two weeks later to have another scan because the twins were quite small and they couldn't check them both, but by the time I went into labour I had at least met my doctor and midwife and discussed the birth. I had a friend who had two-year-old twins, and she lent me some twin books, and I contacted TAMBA (Twins and Multiple Birth Association). At 20 weeks, I had even got in touch with the Wandsworth Twins Club and been to a couple of coffee mornings. It was quite nice to see some babies. It made it a bit more real for me.

'My Mum was seven months pregnant when she found out she was having twins, and she was about three weeks early. My sister had her first baby six weeks early, but I naively thought that everything was going so well with my pregnancy and I felt so well, with no warning contractions or anything, that I might get to term. I thought it would be great to get to 36 weeks, and anything after that would be a bonus. I was eating more, cooking a lot and was quite pleased to eat healthily with a lot of protein and calcium.

'I was made redundant at 20 weeks, so I wasn't working. I had been at home for 10 weeks or so, nesting, having a little nap and sleeping very well. Because everything was going so well, no-one had discussed the risk of prematurity. I didn't even read the chapters in the books about prematurity because I thought "I am going to hold on to my babies." I hadn't done any preparation like visiting the SCBU [special care baby unit, pronounced "skiboo"], and we were due to go for our first NCT class and take a hospital tour the week after they were actually born.

'The labour was very quick. It was a Friday night, after 10pm, and I felt really tired so I said to Jim, who'd just come back from the pub, "I'm feeling a little bit uncomfortable and can't go to sleep." I started wanting to go to the loo a lot, trotting in and out all the time, and at midnight I said "I don't feel quite right." Still not suspecting that this was labour, Jim rang the hospital explaining, "She's 31-weeks pregnant, expecting twins," and they told us to come straight in.

'By then I was starting to have the contractions, and they were coming closer together. They were 10 minutes apart by the time the cab arrived. But we weren't sure whether they were contractions. So I got out of the cab and walked straight into delivery. We arrived at about 1.40am. I handed over my notes and told them what was happening, and I said to the doctor on call, "Am I having the babies?" and he said, "You are definitely having them because you are 5cm dilated."

'I'd had no pain relief, and they put me on my back on the delivery bed. Harry was born at 2.22am and Thomas at 2.32am. Thomas was breech so they tried to turn him around, but couldn't. It was quite scary because it was all so quick. They were keeping the warm cushions and the incubator ready. I had a quick cuddle of Harry and Thomas after they were born. They were both breathing okay, and I felt we were in good hands.

'Jim had a little cuddle and then showed the babies to me. I think they gave Harry to me first while sorting out Tom. Thomas had a little bit more of a struggle to breathe. And then they put them both in the incubators and said they were going off to the special care baby unit, and we were told we could see them whenever we wanted. I think I was in shock. Even though labour was quite short, I felt drained. Surprisingly, the main thing that was hurting me was the salt water (saline) drip, where it went into the back of the hand, so I asked them to take it out. I wasn't shaking or anything, but exhausted. I had a shower and then went to see the babies at around 6am with Jim.

'It was all a bit surreal visiting them. The SCBU was quite a small room and dimly lit. There were about eight or ten incubators and lots of nurses, because it is one-to-one care. The whole room was very warm. It was quite emotional and the consultant said, "The two things you probably want to know are 'are they going to be alright, and when are they going to come home'." He said, "You've got two healthy little babies and the main problem is that they are small. Plan on them coming home on or around their due date – anything else will be a bonus."

'Thomas was on a respirator that first day, so it was a bit traumatic. He was quite bruised and he had a black eye from the birth.

'I was allowed to recover in a single room on the labour ward, which was quite nice except I didn't have my babies and everyone else did. The nurses came up to talk about the feeding quite soon after the birth. And I did feel as though this was my bit to try and help the babies. I'd be there at the hospital about eight hours every day and Jim would join me at midday. I stayed in four nights. Feeding-wise, I would express in the hospital for an hour, 20 minutes per breast, and then express every three to four hours. I had a Modela electric breast pump for the evenings and the mornings. I liked to help feed them by putting the breast milk into the nasal tubes.

'I tried to be really positive when letting close friends and family know, and my Mum was saying prayers for the boys. I think because ours were the biggest in there, and you think "our babies are doing so much better than some of the really small babies in there who are only 25 weeks old" that you no longer think they look so small in the unit.

'They were sleeping all the time. They were always next to each other, although not together. They did put them in cots together after all the wires and drips were taken off. It is nice to get to know what they are filling in on the charts, and they explained all of that. Just before they were allowed home, they put them together. We could stroke them and take them out and cuddle them for short periods.

'My only advice would be to err on the side of caution if you think you might be in labour, and don't be persuaded by anyone else because I think most premature labours are, like mine, quite quick.'

Thanks to research in America, where the number of pre-term babies jumped by 27 per cent between 1981 and 2001, we now know for certain how good the long-term prospects for early babies are. A new study published in the *Journal of the American Medical Association* in February 2003 found that many babies born before 37 weeks 'defy expectations, dramatically improving their mental capacity as they grow'. The study traced the progress of 300 of the smallest babies, including two out of four quads who weighed 11lb in total at birth. In one picture-vocabulary test for children aged between three and eight, they found the scores of the premature babies jumped 11 points, compared to a typical 4.5 jump in non-preemies. Even IQ scores, traditionally believed to be constant during a person's lifetime, had similar jumps – many of those with low IQs (between 70 and 80) at three years of age had normal scores five years later.

Perhaps less explicable with scientific tests, but more understandable on a human level, is how the extra attention given to preemies during their early years seems to benefit their progress as individuals later in life. In a similar fashion, mothers of prem twins seem to be the most successful breastfeeders at coffee mornings, because of all the extra support they receive around the birth; the babies, too, seem to benefit from their doting environment. The study even tracked a group of preemies until they reached the age of 20, and found they were less likely than full-term babies to take up risky behaviour such as drinking, drugs and sex.[3]

Still on the subject of drinking, drugs and sex, you may be interested in hearing of one of the best ways of stopping premature labour once it has started – a glass of wine. America's leading midwife Ina May Gaskin, who helped hundreds of hippy mothers give birth to their babies in 1960s buses on the trail, swears by it and explains why in her book *Spiritual Midwifery* (Book Publishing Company).

'If there has been no bloody show and there is no or very little dilation of the cervix (less than 1cm), give the woman a full glass of water followed by a glass of wine. Alcohol is a depressant, and it suppresses the release of oxytocin from the pituitary gland. It works well for stopping labor in the third trimester. Alcohol should not be used in the first two trimesters to inhibit labor because of possible damage to the developing baby. The woman should stay in bed and everything should be as nice and quiet around her as possible. Making love tends to start rushes [contractions] if a woman is on the edge of starting labor, so the couple should abstain a while in favor of "cooking" their baby a little longer.'

One mother in her book who went into labour at six months managed to cook the baby for a further two months by sipping on vodka when a contraction came and staying in bed. I can think of worse ways to spend the day.

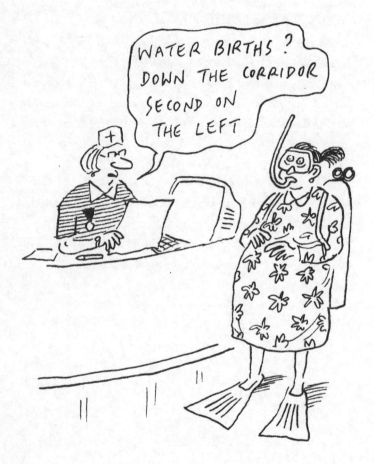

SEVEN

Everything You Want to Know about Twin Birth (and Are Too Afraid to Ask)

As someone who managed to birth her twins naturally, and there will be plenty of you out there who may not have the choice, may I make a quick plug for its benefits. The less medical interference around the birth, the quicker the recovery afterwards. Not forsaking the safety of the babies, if you can deliver them with as little intervention as possible, you will avoid all the side-effects that high-tech obstetrics have on a flesh-and-blood woman. You will also feel as if you have run a marathon, built the Great Wall of China and conquered Everest – all of which sets you up nicely for the next few months. After the triumphant natural delivery of not one but two babies, you will wake up the next day on the most tremendous hormonal high with your body feeling spookily back to normal. Emerging victorious from such a birth will make the night feeds seem like a doddle.

If that's the best we can aim for with a twin birth, it may not be what all of us achieve. Even writing about natural birth implies there might be some competitive element to it, that if you don't cross the finishing line in a certain way, you have somehow failed. **Failure should be the first thing to banish from your mind.** All of us are descended from genetically successful women who have been reproducing for centuries to get us here. There are benefits to a natural birth – a hormonal high better than any drug, a quicker recovery, easier initial bonding, fewer health complications for the mother – but whether you get one or not may not be up to you. Don't set yourself up for disappointment. As long as you do all your homework, and are happy in the knowledge that you have done all you can to give the babies the best possible entrance into the world, then you have already proved that you are a good enough mother. I know you will think about your birth in terms of your babies, so forgive me if I take on the responsibility of thinking about it in terms of you.

First-timers

There are plenty of advantages to having your twins first, before any other children. One twin mother smugly set these out in black and white in our local newsletter:

1. Shopping – you have the great excuse of getting everything new and matching rather than having to buy or borrow one extra.
2. Husbands have no precedent set with a first child so they have no excuse for not being hands on.
3. The first six weeks have to be easier without a toddler around.

But before you congratulate yourself too heartily on the cleverness of your fertility, there is one big mystery you have yet to explore, and that is birth.

You have probably taken your label of 'high risk' that all twin mothers are called in this country, and are wearing it as a badge of pride – hoping for a little more attention as a result. You may even like double the number of scans and the extra fuss that is made when you go in for your pre-natal checkups. You are almost definitely wedded to the idea of a hospital birth, unaware that anything else is even possible. And you may have been told, as I was, that due to the presentation of your babies you should deliver by vaginal and Caesarean (some doctors don't like you to go through labour unless both babies are presented head down) or planned Caesarean.

Whatever you have been told, it is important to believe that you still have choices and, most importantly, that until your babies are born, you have some control. One of the most bewildering aspects of modern birth is that women who are used to making decisions often feel frighteningly out of control. There is plenty you can do to make sure you feel listened to and included every step of the way.

If this is your first birth, of course you do not know how labour and birth will progress on the day, but there is still plenty you can do to plan for it. For you the hardest thing will be knowing what you want, when you have no idea how your body will react. Here are a few things you can do to research your prognosis offered by your doctors, and to make sure that everything goes as smoothly as possible on the day:

- Find out from your mother or sisters how their births went, and what they would have liked to have done to have made them better. We have a peculiar genetic tendency to emulate the birth experiences of our mothers and siblings. My mother told me at a crucial time, when labour was failing to progress with the twins, that she had exactly the same problem when expecting her twins, until the midwife finally broke her waters. I told my midwives this information mid-labour, who then transferred me to hospital to break my waters. The twins were both born within the next 40 minutes.

- Find out from your doctor how they expect the babies to be delivered. Ask whether they are committed to natural childbirth, skilled in turning a breech twin to a head-first position (external version) and what their rate of Caesareans is. Make some notes so you can discuss the answers with the midwives.

- Meet the community midwives. Community midwives are responsible for home births and for looking after mothers when they come out of hospital. They will be responsible for your care in conjunction with the hospital, and may come to your house to take your blood samples during pregnancy. Discuss the doctor's prognosis for birth and ask them to give suggestions about how to help it go well on the day.

- Meet the hospital midwives. They are separate from the community midwives although occasionally you may find one of your community midwives in the ward. Ask to be shown a twin delivery suite (they often have extra monitoring equipment to the normal delivery suite). Ask the hospital midwives how you could decorate the delivery suite on the day to make yourself feel more comfortable (the extra equipment sometimes means that the suite is lacking in the normal flowery curtains and jolly wall pictures that other rooms have). Ask to meet any of the hospital midwives experienced in twin delivery and make a note of their names for the future.

- Join your local NCT (National Childbirth Trust) class. NCT classes start around 30 weeks but you can use your 'twins come early' excuse to join one a little sooner if you want to become more informed about your birth. Ask the leader of the NCT class if she knows of any twin mothers in the class that had good births and who might be available for a chat.

- Write a birth plan (*see below*). Doctors respond well to pieces of paper, particularly if they are typed. Using the letter I wrote to my doctor as a template, ask the doctor to go through the birth plan with you, commenting on their own particular hospital procedures. This way you will know what to expect and will have fewer surprises on the day. Doctors tend to focus on problems, rather than positives, so always ask them 'and what is the best-case scenario to expect?'

- Choose a keen birth partner. If your husband isn't that keen to be your 'labour coach', rather than force him, consider who might be a good alternative. Sometimes the presence of another woman who had a good birth herself, like a girlfriend or your mother, can be tremendously reassuring. Your husband will be on hand for the main moment, but labour can last a long time, and there may be room for others to share in supporting you (this can also leave the husband a little more refreshed to take over when the babies are born). Whoever you choose, the more visits to NCT classes and the hospital the birth partner makes with you, the more familiar they are with the transfer to hospital on the day. If you want extra professional support, think about paying for an independent midwife (*see below*).

- Look forward to it. It may seem weirdly masochistic to say that pain is only a part of birth. 'Pain with a purpose' or 'positive pain', if such phrases existed, is quite different from the stubbing-your-toe sort. We women are better equipped to deal with pain than our partners, and you will have so many hormones swilling around you on the day that you may be as cool as a cucumber while everyone around you is burning their fingers on the hot water and towels. Enjoy the fuss. A woman in labour is a queen bee. Soon enough, you will be elbowed sideways for others to get a better view of the babies.

- Pack a bag for the big day. If this helps you feel more excited rather than fearful, pack up your hospital bag with all those shopping extras that you find on the Boots shelves. Fizzy glucose drinks, favourite snacks, weeny babygros, newborn nappies all ready packed for D-day. Ignore the doomsayers that say they are superstitious about buying anything until after the birth; you want only to be surrounded with positive people and happy thoughts about how cute your twins will look in white velour teddy suits.

Second time around

Okay, so you've been through the birth thing once. You know what it is all about and how your body reacts on the day. You may have some inkling about how you want things to be different this time around. (For me, this was remembering huffing and puffing in the last stages of birthing my first son, thinking to myself 'next time I'm getting fit for this'). It may be that this time, because you already have a demanding toddler at home also to think about, you want as little upset to the family as possible. The main thing to know is that whatever your prognosis for birth, there is still plenty you can do to improve on your first-time experience.

For example, if you had a section the first time, and have therefore assumed that the twins will be born the same way, think again. Would you like to try for something different this time, or do you want to repeat what you know? If you don't want to try for a VBAC (vaginal birth after Caesarean), then it may be just a question of choosing your twins' birthday. If you do want to try for a natural birth, you may have to do a bit of extra homework to secure support for your decision – particularly because of the 'high risk' label.

Perhaps the first port of call would be a midwife or doctor who is committed to natural childbirth and experienced enough with natural twin births to want to help you. Your doctor or midwife should inspire you with confidence and have trust in the birth process, so don't be fobbed off with the 'let's see what happens on the day' talk. Natural twin birth is a little more complicated than a single delivery, so a lot will depend very much on where you live and what sort of services are around you. But there is always someone out there who is willing to help. If all else fails, you can always call the wonderful Beverley Beech at the Association of Improvement in Maternity Services (01753 652781; www.aims.org.uk), and she will do her best to find an independent midwife to take on your case.

Know your birth rights

Just by reading your rights as a pregnant woman in the National Health Service, you will enter your next doctor's appointment standing a little bit taller. Or, perhaps later on in labour itself, you might remember one of them and exercise it on the spot.

I know one twin mother who wished on reflection that she had used her rights to ask for a second opinion when her doctor announced that he wanted to perform her Caesarean on Christmas Eve, well before her babies' due date. When she questioned him about the necessity, she was told she was being 'selfish'. It may have suited the doctor to have her case out of the way before he went on his Christmas holidays, but it certainly added to her burden. Now she has to organize two birthdays before the biggest holiday of the year.

As a pregnant woman, you are entitled to the following:[1]

- To opt for midwifery care only.
- A home birth (although this may be difficult to get on the NHS, there are plenty of examples of twin home births using independent midwives).
- To refuse to be attended by anyone you do not wish present, such as a medical student (I politely asked a student to

wait outside for my second doctor's appointment, because at the first, with a student present, I didn't feel I had the doctor's proper attention).

- ◊ A second opinion. (I also tried to change doctors when my own recommended a vaginal birth and Caesarean for my twins).
- ◊ A copy of the research paper that supports the advice you are being given.
- ◊ A copy of the hospital protocol or guidelines for the relevant aspect of your care, such as induction of labour. (I asked for the twin birth protocol from my hospital, and was able to clarify what some of the medical jargon meant with my doctor).
- ◊ To refuse any treatment you do not wish to receive.
- ◊ A copy of your records and the correspondence about your case (free if you apply within 40 days of your last consultation).

These are your rights, so don't be afraid to use them. If you do, your story might help the next twin mother who comes after you and is unaware that she has any. Don't be afraid to challenge the hospital's authority if you are unhappy with what you are being told. It is in the hospital's interest, not yours, to have all of us women herded into a single maternity ward, served by fewer midwives than if we were at home or in a birth centre. And until the babies are born you have plenty of rights to help you make that very un-British thing, a fuss. You are going to have to raise your voice soon enough to get a double trolley at the supermarket, so you might as well get some practice in now.

Know your hospital protocols

It was surprising for me to learn that despite all NHS hospitals using the same cardboard pillowcases and sheets, they all differ in their twin birth protocols. This means that every hospital subscribes to a different code of practice for twins, a piece of paper that may well affect how your birth goes. This paper will not be given to you, but you are quite entitled to a copy. You just have to ask.

For example, the twin birth protocol for my hospital in London stated that 'Under no circumstances was there any place for a natural Third Stage Delivery' (*see glossary on pages 105–6*). This means that unless I had made it clear beforehand that I wanted to deliver the placenta without an injection of drugs, it would have been given to me routinely. Third-stage natural delivery is just a way of letting your body do its thing without yet more interference to speed things up. And you can rest assured that after delivering two babies, delivering the placenta is a cinch.

Personally, I felt a lot of anxiety at the prospect of a Caesarean, especially when I learnt there would be 10 or 12 people present in the theatre, because extra pairs of hands are needed for the twins. Call me private, or someone who suffers from performance anxiety, but this very public spectacle of my birth gave me sleepless nights. I later learnt that this fear of being attended to in labour by strangers is a common one, and only in the West do we make birth into a semi-public spectacle, where any old student nurse or hospital cleaner can attend. In other cultures the 'birth chamber' is always attended by a strictly specified group of people – midwife, female relatives and other women who have borne children – so my fears were deep rooted.

I also worried that a Caesarean would be a greater risk for me, with higher blood loss and potential difficulties with the scar healing. With a vaginal delivery for the first and a section for the second, I was concerned that I would have all the effort of a natural birth with none of the benefits of quick recovery afterwards. As it was, enlisting the services of independent midwives allowed me to labour as I wanted with the second twin being born breech.

Alternatives to the NHS

Independent midwives

If you want some guarantee of a good twin birth, which, after all, is a bit more complicated than your average singleton, I highly recommend you put aside some money to have a professional on your side. Take out some insurance, extend your mortgage or borrow from your parents as I did. I don't regret that extra reassurance, because when push came to shove, if you'll excuse the phrase, and twin two came down the birth canal showing an arm and a leg, I had one of the most experienced midwives in the country, Mary Cronk, to push her back up, put a finger in her mouth and deliver her breech within seconds. I shudder to think what might have happened if those seconds had turned to minutes and my midwife was not there. Paying for independent midwives takes the lottery element out of our NHS system.

The great thing about independent midwives is that I felt I was always being listened to during the process and I felt in charge (if not always in control). My physical and emotional feelings were attended to. I was able to eat and drink to keep up my strength during my long, but not particularly painful, labour because I was being cared for at home. (Often in hospital, you are forbidden food or drink in case you need a general anaesthetic.) I was able to rehearse how the birth would go, and labouring at home meant I was in a familiar environment. When I had to go into the hospital because my labour was not progressing, I did so with my two midwives, whose familiarity, as well as comprehensive notes on my labour so far, helped to make the transfer as easy as possible. How different from the many women whose labour stops on arrival in hospital because they are moved somewhere strange and the hormone adrenalin kicks in.

Minutes after the birth, I took a bath with the two babies. I was tactfully left alone with my husband and our two new arrivals when he came in to meet them, thus ensuring those precious moments of initial bonding were private. I was allowed home immediately, which is what I wanted, and ate my first meal after the birth, bacon and eggs with champagne, in our double bed at home. The first night all four of us slept together, with no cacophony of other babies crying or the impossibility of trying to fit two babies into an NHS single bed. The next day, as I sat in the bath with my newly deflated stomach, I felt strangely normal. Unlike my first birth, I had no backache from the epidural needle, no tearing or episiotomy, nothing that had made my body feel prodded and poked.

If you appoint independent midwives for your twins, you will be ascribed three midwives for the birth – one for each baby and one for you. Because they operate privately, they are likely to have a lot of experience – two of the most experienced in the country are Jane Evans and Mary Cronk. One midwife will be responsible for most of your pre-natal and post-natal care, and they will all visit you daily for 10 days and then continue to visit as much as you require (both of mine attended the twins' first birthday party). Independent midwives tend to birth at home, but sometimes it is possible to organize for them to be attached to a hospital. In any event, should you need to transfer to hospital for any reason – as I did because my labour did not progress – they will come in with you to assist. Having independent midwives costs around £2,500 for twins. For more information, phone 01483 821104, visit www.independentmidwives.org.uk or send an s.a.e. to 1 The Great Quarry, Guildford GU1 3XL.

Birth centre

There is only one proper private birth centre in the UK, and it was set up by the former President of the Royal College of Midwives, Caroline Flint. Unless you live in London, or are prepared to move to London for the birth, however, it may well be out of your geographical area. Providing the rules on insurance have not been changed, you will be treated to the only private practice that can operate within London hospitals. Speaking to the midwife Pam Wild about my options before the twins were due, she told me about twins that had been delivered in water to a first-time mother in Homerton Hospital, East London (with the doctor waiting outside the door and only invited in at the end to congratulate the mother), and a natural triplet birth they assisted in Kings College Hospital, central London.

The Birth Centre is peopled by committed and experienced professionals who are intent on giving you a good birth experience. The cost falls somewhere between £2,500 to £4,000 (no extra for twins), depending on how early in your pregnancy you take up their care. Caroline Flint Midwifery Services can be contacted on 0207 498 2322 or visit their website www.thebirthcentre.co.uk

NHS birth centres are unlikely to take on a mother expecting twins because of the 'high risk' label. However, if you have heard of a good one in your area, there is no reason why you can't give them a call to talk to a midwife about your local NHS options. Birth centres are often peopled by professionals who are keen to offer an alternative to the medicalized hospital route.

Private hospitals

If you have health insurance that covers you for pregnancy, or have the means to birth your twins privately, you may want to consider a private hospital. In the UK, the private hospitals are all found in London, and those that deliver twins include the Portland Hospital, St Mary's Hospital (Lindo Wing), Queen Charlotte's Hospital and Chelsea and Westminster (St John and St Elizabeth Hospital – the celeb's choice – sadly does not).

Some of these private hospitals, such as Chelsea and Westminster, subscribe to the same twin birth protocols as the NHS hospitals, and are really more of a 'lifestyle option' of cosier rooms than an alternative birth option. Others such as Queen Charlotte's (also the home of the Multiple Birth Foundation) describe themselves as 'consultancy-led', and therefore your birth options will be between you and whichever of the five consultants you choose. If your insurance company is picking up the bill, then the breakdown of figures you get may not look so daunting. If not, expect to pay around £3,250 to £4,000 for the consultant's charge, an anaesthetist's charge of £275 to £350 for an epidural, plus between £831 to £1,240 for your first 24 hours' care (after that it is £324 per night). Scans and consultant paediatricians come as extra.

BIG WORDS DOCTORS USE ABOUT LABOUR AND BIRTH

Dilating/dilation. This describes the opening of the cervix in readiness for the baby to come down the birth canal. The measurement used is in centimetres, so you will be described as '2cm dilated' in very early labour, or '7cm dilated' when well on the way, with the jackpot being '10 cm dilated' – big enough to accommodate a baby's head.

First stage. This is early labour. The contractions may be coming but in between you are able to talk, move around, have a bath and eat. Your cervix is opening slowly (or quickly), depending on how your body behaves.

Second stage. Often described as 'the desire to push', this stage can be relatively short compared to the first stage. It starts when you are fully dilated and the baby is ready to be born. The transition from first stage to second stage can be quite subtle, and an experienced midwife should be able to recognize it (the transition is sometimes marked by the mother becoming fed up and tired, complaining that she can't go on any more).

Third stage. Pushing out the afterbirth, or to use the technical term, expelling the placenta. It seems a bit of a drag that you have yet another job to do after having the two babies, but your body will do it for you with just a few mini-contractions. Some hospitals routinely give an injection of syntocin to hurry things along. Don't forget to insist on a natural third-stage delivery early on, if you want it.

Apgar score. This is the test they perform on newborns for pinkness and alertness. Traditionally, the second twin has a lower apgar score on birth than the first twin because they have been hanging around waiting for their sibling to be born first. This is quite normal. Most babies 'pink up nicely' even if their apgar scores are a little low on delivery. The traditionally lower apgar score for the second twin is the reason why some doctors (unnecessarily) suggest a Caesarean, as the *British Medical Journal* reported in the November 2002 edition.

Birth plan for natural birth

If you are sure you want a natural birth, it is a good idea to state your commitment in a letter to your doctor that may also double as a birth plan. Using the American reference book *Having Twins* by Elizabeth Noble (*see Further Reading*),

I wrote the following document for discussion with my doctor. It was useful, and although in the end we opted for independent midwife-only care, it did help us clarify exactly what support we would receive from the NHS. The doctor's comments on the birth plan are written in parentheses.

18 November 2000

Birth plan for twins for:
Emma A.G. Barker
Hospital no: 01170811

Dear doctors, paediatricians and midwives who may be attendant at delivery,

Please find below the requests of my husband Adam and I for labour, delivery and the immediate post-partum period at Chelsea and Westminster Hospital. My husband Adam and I are keen for me to have as little medical intervention as possible during labour and delivery in order to bond with and nurse the babies immediately after birth, and to leave the hospital as soon as we are deemed fit to do so.

We are well aware of the complications of a twin delivery. We have read your hospital guidelines for the management of twin delivery and spoken to professionals and parents who have delivered twins naturally.

While we trust your medical judgment and feel confident that you will support our requests as long as they are medically feasible, we would be most grateful if you would raise any points in the plan that you feel are unacceptable or inadmissible at this early stage.

Our requests include those for a 'natural' birth and those for one with complications. Both assume that labour will not be induced early, and that I will be allowed to go full term plus, as my mother did when she was carrying my brother and I as twins.

Requests in the Event of a Normal Birth

1. To labour in a pool in the hospital at the beginning of active labour (here the doctor wrote, 'if less than 2–3 cm dilated; in active labour I would advise monitoring of both twins').
2. To be attended by my husband Adam.
3. To be attended by midwives only – at least one midwife experienced in twin birth overseeing the labour (the doctor wrote 'understands may not be available').
4. To have no interns or students observing the birth.
5. To have no routine prep – shaving or enema (doctor explained this no longer happens in hospitals any more).
6. To have access to gas and air as the only form of tranquillizer or pain medication.
7. To have no routine stimulants to start or speed up labour.

8. To have no routine rupture of membranes.
9. To have no routine intravenous drip.
10. To have no routine electronic foetal-heart monitoring but to use a hand-held sonicaid to monitor (doctor underlined 'routine' and wrote 'not routine, but because twins are high risk').
11. To be free to walk around during labour – no routine confinement to bed or the labour room.
12. To be taken to the delivery room with the experienced midwife in attendance.
13. To have the option to modify delivery positions: for example, not to use stirrups or cuffs, to deliver on my side, hands and knees, squatting, standing up – whatever position feels comfortable at the time – for the first and second baby.
14. If possible for Adam to receive the first baby to say 'hello' immediately after s/he is born. We do not want the baby put into a warmer – or given straight to a paediatrician for inspection. Likewise, Adam and I should also have the opportunity to receive the second baby. If possible, I would like to nurse one or both immediately. [One of the most common complaints from triplet mothers is that their babies are taken away immediately for inspection. This is often quoted as their only regret about the birth.]
15. If the breech takes more than the hospital guidelines of 20 minutes and the heart rate of the second baby is normal, labour of second baby to be allowed to progress with no rush for as long as mother and supporting midwife allow. This may be anything up to or over an hour.[2]

16. To allow for a physiological third stage of labour. No injections of Ergometrine or infusion of syntocin or syntometrine unless mother agrees.
17. To prevent excess blood loss and complications in the third stage, to allow the cord of the first twin to cease pulsating before clamping and separation, and also to allow the second twin's cord to cease pulsating before interference (the doctor ticked this request).

Requests in the Event of Complications During Labour and Delivery

1. For the obstetrician to meet the above requests if medically feasible.
2. If I should have to have a Caesarean birth, to have Adam present so that he can hold the babies to begin the bonding process.

Requests to the Paediatrician if One or Both Babies Require Care in the Special Care Unit

1. To be able to hold the babies, if medically feasible, or at least touch them before they go to the Special Care Baby Unit.
2. To have the babies receive breast milk that I pump for them and to nurse as soon as they are able.

For discussion: whether in addition to my husband, Adam, I would be able to bring in a birth attendant familiar with the birthing process.

Thank you for taking the time to review and discuss these requests.

Yours sincerely,

Emma Barker
Adam Barker

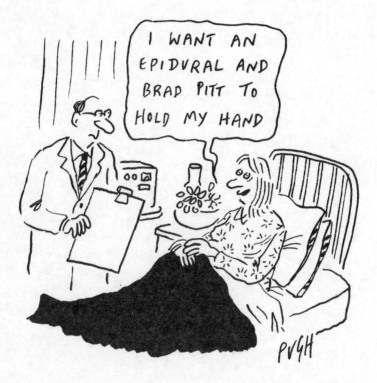

EIGHT

Ready for D-Day

If you are reading this and your stomach feels like a seething mass of limbs, and your body like a double for the *Alien*, then you may already be fantasizing about being induced. Those last weeks of a twin pregnancy throw new light on the old-fashioned term 'confinement'. You don't feel like going out because even a casual stroll seems fraught with pavement danger when you can't see your feet. Or perhaps you cannot face people looking sympathetic at your one-woman freak show (I attempted a swim in my last week, and a young girl shouted across the pool 'Mummy, Mummy – look at that lady over there! Just look how *fat* she is!').

Classes, clubs and coffee mornings

There is good reason to use the universal assumption of 'twins coming early' to take that extra time off work to pamper yourself well before the babies are due. This may be the last time for a year that you get to put your feet up properly without remembering some little job of sterilizing bottles or buying nappies, so go ahead and lie down. **After all, you are always at work, making two babies, not one.** Who else in the office can boast the same?

Twins clubs

There is one worthwhile destination at this late stage of the game, and that is a local twins club coffee morning. If you haven't already joined, and even if you are sceptical about clubs, this could prove to be an important fact-finding mission. If not, just the act of cooing over someone else's newborn twins while munching on chocolate biscuits amounts to a good day of maternity leave. Call before you attend a coffee morning, and usually the host mother will ring around for others at a similar stage to you to come along. You will be amazed at how you find yourself bursting with the sort of questions that immediately slip your mind when faced with a doctor.

Antenatal classes

Antenatal classes are another must for new mothers. They start in the 30th week of pregnancy, lasting for eight weeks. If you are keen to start earlier, you can always use that universal excuse again of twins coming early to fit in with your own plans. The National Childbirth Trust (NCT) ones are easily the best, and contrary to some people's opinion, will not insist that you give birth naturally in a swimming pool wafting joss sticks and playing whale music. Jo Sweeney, the helpline co-ordinator at the NCT, says 'We don't advocate a particular course of action but try to inform women of their wider options.' The NCT will often put an expectant twin mother in touch with a mother of newborn twins who has had a good birth experience. Call the NCT helpline to find out where your local classes are held (0870 444 8707).

Hospitals also hold their own antenatal classes, although you won't be having the same cosy get-together after the birth as you will with your NCT lot. My own hospital antenatal classes are credited with putting my husband Adam off the maternity ward for life. The welcome evening included an X-rated video called *Stephanie's labour*, complete with real groans from the delivery suite. As the lights went up, I sighed and turned to Adam, only to find that he had left the building for 20 cigarettes. You have been warned.

More useful might be the special antenatal classes that are being developed around the country by the Twins and Multiple Birth Association (TAMBA 0870 770 3305). By the time you read this, classes should be underway with specific information on birthing more than one baby. **TAMBA is also the place to call to find out how to contact your local twins club.** Subscriptions to TAMBA and a local twins club cost only a few quid. For up-to-date details on talks and seminars, visit www.tamba.org.uk (don't forget the 'uk' or you will become an expert on West African drumming).

Similarly, the Multiple Births Foundation (MBF: 0208 383 3519) holds useful Prenatal Evenings for families expecting twins, as well as offering free literature at Queen Charlotte's in Hammersmith, West London.

Nesting, nesting, one, two, three

Fortunately, nature is kind to us women at the end of pregnancy by softening our brains. So even though you are waddling very slowly through doorways and constantly catching your buttons on handles, you also have no desire whatsoever to visit an art gallery, attend the Harrods sale or go out to a nightclub. Despite a hundred years of feminism, hormones still triumph, and a pregnant mother of twins has nothing more important on her mind than nappy systems and moving the furniture around.

So, the last few weeks are the time to use your massive size and vulnerability to get in other people to 'nest' on your behalf. If an odd-job man does not fix that leaking kitchen tap, it will not get fixed for another six months. If you don't get your windows professionally cleaned tomorrow, you will see their smeariness in all the photos. With twins, you have the perfect excuse – and built-in urgency – to get jobs done for you. I even pulled the twin pregnancy number in a mobile phone shop, when I was told that I had to take the handset to another store. 'But my doctor told me that I could give birth at any moment and I need it NOW.' A phone call later and a new handset was handed over, and the door held open. Use it while you can. Doors will soon swing shut on your double buggy when the bump is gone.

For God's sake, give me some drugs

There is much to be said for thinking about pain relief before the big day, maybe even trying a puff on the gas and air if your antenatal classes allow it. It seems a bit hard on labouring women to try all these new drugs on a day when they have so much else to think about, particularly as many of us react better to some than to others.

The interesting thing about pain is that perception of pain – the expectation of something hurting like hell – is far worse than the reality of it. When you consider that **the worst contraction on earth lasts no longer than a minute**, and that in between two contractions you will be able to joke with the midwife, it makes the business of birth seem less frightening.

As well as contractions, there is the 'crowning of the head', when the widest part of the head comes out of the birth canal, also affectionately known as the 'ring of fire'. Scared yet? Don't be. Yes, it hurts like hell, but it only lasts for a matter of seconds. Once it is all over, the pain is forgotten.

What makes childbirth so different from any other sort of pain is that it is **pain with a purpose**. No other pain produces heavenly beings afterwards. And once the first twin has done all the work, the second baby should be plain sailing down the birth canal. If you are still unconvinced whether you can handle it, remember that all that huffing and puffing, sweating and swearing does wonders for the skin.

Here is what the medical establishment currently doles out if you shout for it. Just don't confuse pain relief with anaesthetic. One helps you manage your own pain; the other takes away your control.

Tens machine

This never worked for me. I found it was like having an annoying transistor radio attached to my side. The machine works by deflecting the body's attention away from the pain of a contraction by issuing electronic impulses which can be increased manually, like turning up the volume on a stereo, as the contraction increases. The concept is rather like digging your nails into the palm of your hand to distract from the pain elsewhere. They can be hired from Boots and other chemists, and have the advantage of being tried out ahead of time. Many people swear by Tens machines, and can manage the whole of their labour pain on it. Mine was ripped off early on with a plea for something more hardcore.

Entonox – gas and air

This involves sucking on a tube, or inhaling through a mouthpiece, to take the edge off a contraction. It definitely makes you a little high, which is an advantage or disadvantage depending on what floats your boat. Some, like me, love it. Others, like my friend Rikke, didn't. She likened it to smoking a joint. The technique with gas and air is to start sucking on the mouthpiece as soon as you feel the contraction starting, so that at the peak of the contraction you have taken in enough of the stuff to ride the wave.

It has no after effects; the feeling-woozy sensation goes away immediately. Gas and air is available for home births.

Epidural or spinal block

This is anaesthesia administered from the waist downwards. It is particularly useful for 'back' labours, when the baby's spine is opposite to your own and labour is that much more difficult and painful. This was the case for my firstborn, and after a long labour that wasn't progressing, it worked a treat, allowing me to relax and progress from 5cm to 10cm dilation in 20 minutes. The downside is that, unless you have a mobile epidural, you are stuck on the bed and prone to medical intervention – starting with an intravenous drip to speed up your contractions and ending with an episiotomy (snip). Also, you are on your back, and therefore unable to adopt the best position for birthing – on your hands and knees. The after-effects, apart from feeling run over by a bus from all the medical interference, is a nagging backache for weeks where the needle was inserted. Not everyone has this, but most women complain of backache afterwards.

Pethidine

This morphine derivative is rarely used these days but can be used for home births along with gas and air (an epidural needs a skilled anaesthetist to administer it in hospital). I've always wanted to try pethidine, but it is not so popular these days because the drug crosses the placenta and can make the baby drowsy. Despite this, my midwife Mary Cronk says that her notes from 20 years ago showed substantially larger doses given to mothers than today, with good outcomes for the mothers and babies.

Syntocin

This synthetic form of oxytocin, the main hormone that stimulates the uterus to contract, is given via an intravenous drip. It is sometimes used to bring on labour artificially as an alternative to breaking the bag of waters (when waters are broken, it is usually recommended that a baby is delivered within 72 hours to prevent infection). Syntocin may also be given to speed up labour and after the babies' delivery to stimulate the womb to deliver the placenta.

Am I in labour?

This may seem like a stupid question to ask, but don't be surprised if you find this your mantra as the pregnancy wears on. Somehow we are expected to know whether or not we are in labour, as if a host of angels will suddenly serenade you to the labour ward to announce you are officially giving birth. The reality is somewhat different. Take the mother who insisted on being driven immediately to the hospital because her waters had broken in the car, only to find on arrival that she was 'still pregnant' and had been sitting on a wet car seat after her husband had mistakenly left the car window open in the rain.

Take also the fact that 'early', 'latent' or even 'false labour' as it used to be called can mean that you are having contractions five minutes apart, but the contractions are only positioning the baby, or getting their lungs used to the idea of breathing. Of course, on the other side of the fence, you may be one of those two-pushes-and-they-were-out sort, who specializes in super-quick deliveries.

For this reason, labour is often referred to as 'active labour' when things are really starting to move. But be aware that early labour can involve tightenings which feel like contractions SEVERAL DAYS before you are actually in labour (four in my case). You feel excited and don't rest well (birth hormones are adrenalin-based and become more active) and are absolutely certain that you are in labour (whether you've had a baby or not). However, **one thing is for certain: you will not be in labour unless the whole business is progressing.** Labour is about progress, the inexorable movement towards the ultimate goal – the body producing a baby. Anything that 'goes off' or 'quietens down' is just limbering up.

This is worth knowing because, if you didn't, you might just wear yourself out before your help is finally needed (pushing, my dear). **What you should be doing is eating well, drinking lots of fluid and resting, resting, resting.** What you are probably doing is running all over the house saying, 'I know I put my maternity pants somewhere, why isn't anybody helping?'

If you can bear it, and the midwives agree, stay at home for as long as possible. Go for walks, have lovely baths, ask a friend to come over and make you peanut butter and Marmite sandwiches but try not to whizz into hospital on the first contraction. Unless you are fearful of being at home for some reason, labour progresses much better when you are relaxed and in your own environment, not hooked up to monitors like the bride of Frankenstein.

Finally, when in active labour at home, keep asking yourself, as if it's your birthday, 'what do I want to do now?' and do it. If you are desperate to do something, but can't think what it is, repeat the following affirmation: **'To birth well I must give myself fully to the task but I also must let go and "let it happen by itself". Women who birth well control their surrender to the process. Birth is learning to control surrender.'** Repeat after me, **'Birth is learning to control surrender.'**

Physical signs of early labour

Waters breaking

This can either be a small trickle coming from a tear in the amniotic sac or a sudden gush (one mother describes bending down for a tin of baked beans in the supermarket, followed by 'splashdown!'). Remember, however, that your waters might not break (officially known as 'rupture of membranes') until you are in established labour, and occasionally babies are born in their amniotic sac (*see Julie's birth story on pages 128–32*). When your waters do break, you should tell your midwives immediately. Hospitals might want to monitor your progress and have the babies delivered within the next 72 hours to prevent infection.

Contractions

Another sign of early labour is when contractions come 10 minutes apart or less, have been going on for at least an hour, and are getting stronger or more frequent.

Mucus plug

A glob of period-like stuff that looks just like it sounds. The plug can appear some days before labour starts because the cervix has begun to open and thin out. A 'show' is an old-fashioned term for the passage of the mucus plug, resulting in a blood-stained pair of underpants.

OTHER POSSIBLE PHYSICAL SIGNS OF EARLY LABOUR

- Nagging or intermittent backache
- Diarrhoea
- Feeling nauseous or flu-like
- Increased vaginal discharge
- Nesting instinct – sudden desire to clean the top of the wardrobe or sort out your underwear drawer (not a reliable indicator for tidy freaks)

Women who birth well

According to the handout[1] given to me by my independent midwife, Annie Francis, all women who birth well do the same things and can explain the following about themselves to others. Remember, all these traits are learned behaviour, not inherited, so there is still time to practise the following.

Women who birth well:

1. Breathe effectively and in a relaxed manner.
2. Use their breath to renew themselves with an inhalation and to reduce tension with an exhalation through nose or mouth.
3. Use their breath as a focus.
4. Are aware of how to maintain and recapture relaxation in the inside of their bodies.
5. Maintain a body posture which facilitates the experience and helps the baby descend through the body.
6. Are internally aware and can explain what is happening either while in labour or afterwards.
7. Touch themselves appropriately to facilitate their experience.
8. Help others to know how to assist them.
9. Make certain they go into labour rested.
10. Focus their mental capacity to the task at hand and let other things sit on the side until a more appropriate time.
11. Focus moment to moment. They do not dwell on the past or future of the experience.

12. Say 'I know what I am doing' and 'I manage myself well'.
13. Say 'If I lost it for a moment, I got back on track'.

To this I would add, 'have a sense of humour'. If you can laugh in between contractions and through your labour, that is the best relaxation technique of all.

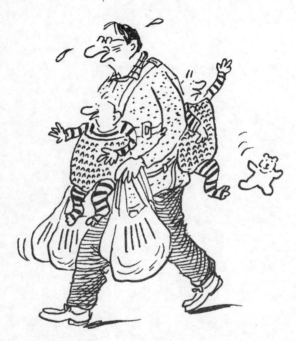

NINE

Happy Birth Days

Your bag is packed, you have raided your CD collection for your favourite soft music, you have a stack of *Hello!* magazines in the side pockets (although you know that the picture captions will be taxing at this stage) and you are waiting for your waters to break. You have read the 'Am I in Labour?' section in the last chapter a dozen times to check whether you have missed anything, and whenever you feel a kick from inside you wonder whether it might be a contraction. Fear of the unknown, excitement that it will soon be over, worry that it will go okay, exhaustion from not being able to sleep properly and relief that your body will soon be your own again are just a few of the emotions roller-coastering around you in this period. And on top of it all, there is a nagging suspicion that these babies may be a lot easier to deal with inside your stomach than outside.

Well, before I dissolve into clichés about how all births are different, let me just demonstrate the point by giving you birth stories of different twins born in different ways. **All of**

them are 'good' birth stories with happy outcomes, so don't feel you have to read them peeking through cracks in your fingers.

First-time-around mothers

'I just followed my own intuition and was lucky enough to get what I wanted.'

Julie, 30, had her non-identical twins naturally in September 2002, assisted by the private independent midwife Mary Cronk. They were her first children and, despite some concerns about her blood pressure, she didn't want to spend time in hospital. Her story is related here by the midwife Mary Cronk [with square brackets of explanation supplied by me where needed].

'My client had engaged my services when 16 weeks into her first pregnancy. She explained that she did not intend to have any ultrasound or screening tests, and intended to give birth at home. She was healthy, intelligent, informed, and I hoped I could assist her to birth her baby as she intended. I laid my hand on her tum. This was either a 20-week pregnancy, or more than one baby. We discussed dates. The couple were pretty sure when this baby had been started so we decided it was likely to be twins. We discussed a scan to confirm. 'Why?' asked Julie, 'surely it will become evident as the pregnancy progresses?' Quite right, I thought. I am not that bad at palpation [feeling the babies] that I can't feel three poles later in this pregnancy [poles are the head and bottom of the baby – if there are more than two then it must be twins]. The pregnancy progressed and Julie and I became more convinced that this was twins.

'We did, however, decide on a scan, not only to confirm the presence of twins but also to find out whether we had monochorionic [one outer sac] or dichorionic [two outer sac] twins. We thought this important as the information would change the advice I gave and the management of the pregnancy. The scan showed dichorionic [two outer sacs] twins growing nicely (which we knew anyway) and two placentae.

'We planned a home birth and I organized that two other midwives would be available for the births. We discussed why a hospital birth might become a better option and Julie shared with me her real fear and dislike of hospitals and their 'procedures'. She had really found attending for the scan very difficult and asked me not to mention the 'H' word again. I was mainly concerned about pregnancy-induced hypertension (PIH) [high blood pressure] as Julie had a double whammy in that she was a primigravida (first-time mother) and twinning. I discussed the case with my supervisor, who was supportive. Julie's BP (blood pressure) was 110/60 at booking and it stayed around that level until 36–37 weeks when, quite suddenly, it rose accompanied by oedema [accumulation of fluid in the tissues of the body, causing swelling]. By 37 weeks, her BP was 140/90 and she had increasing oedema. Julie was doing all the right things, eating a high-protein diet with lots of fruit and veg. She and her husband were professional organic gardeners so it was all good stuff. She was also resting but with some gentle exercise.

'That evening, her blood pressure continued rising and the oedema increased. She was symptom-free – no headache, abdominal pain or visual disturbances. I strongly advised hospital admission and Julie agreed to this. However, she discharged herself the next day as she felt exhausted by lack of sleep and very hungry as the hospital diet was not to her liking (surprise, surprise!). So there she was at home, not quite 38 weeks, babies seemed to be growing nicely, plenty of liquor [fluid in the amniotic sacs, not drinks cabinet], and both babies sounded happy. The only cause for concern was her PIH. I did a vaginal examination at her request and found a head nicely in the pelvis. We hoped for labour. I gave Julie 30ml of castor oil to swallow [caster oil should only be given to pregnant women under a midwife's supervision] but over the next three days there was no labour. Her blood pressure stayed up, her oedema got worse and the blood picture was deteriorating [the results of the blood tests showed the presence of pre-eclampsia]. Although the babies stayed happy, I didn't.

'During her short stay in hospital, Julie had been prescribed Labetelol [a blood pressure-lowering drug which does not treat the underlying PIH] and she also had a scan that showed both babies head down. The reason why a hospital birth might have been my choice is that, in cases of PIH, there are risks to the mother of fits, and there is also a small risk of her having a stroke, and heavy blood loss due to low platelet count. Had either of these unlikely things happened during the labour, medical help would have been more quickly available in a hospital setting.

'Anyway, Julie made a well-informed choice to stay at home and we awaited events. Her BP did come down a bit on Labetelol. She consulted an acupuncturist and had three treatments to treat the PIH and to encourage labour. I did yet another 'stretch and sweep' [to stimulate the cervix to produce prostaglandin] and had never felt a more ripe cervix.

'Monday morning at 6.25 my phone rang. Her husband said Julie's waters had broken and she was having strong pains. I leapt from my bed into my clothes and into the car, arriving at Julie's home at 7.10am. While driving, I called my partner Andrea and asked her to join me. Our planned third midwife was unavailable and Andrea was an hour's drive away so I phoned the hospital labour ward, spoke to the supervisor of midwives on duty and asked for help.

'When I arrived, Julie was on all-fours, obviously in strong labour, having frequent, strong contractions. Five minutes after my arrival, I was joined by the labour ward coordinator who had been on duty all night but had come to assist me. I could have kissed her! Julie's BP was 150/95 [the normal range is from 100/60 to 135/85] and both foetal hearts were fine. I quickly got the room – the downstairs sitting room – set up and two baby resuscitation stations ready with two bags and masks and two warm pads. The labour was obviously progressing well and rapidly.

'At 8am, Andrea arrived, and I could have kissed her too. So the three of us quickly decided who would do what. Julie started to push spontaneously and there were signs of full dilation with both foetal hearts okay. Julie remained on all fours and was coping superbly. At 8.45, I saw the birth of the first beautiful baby, born in the membranes [the waters for this baby never broke, she was born in a full amniotic sac – considered very lucky in the old days]. The membranes were wiped off her face and she was in good nick. We helped Julie pick her baby up. 'Oh my Gawd. I've done it! Its a girl!' she said.

'At 9am, Julie and her husband were admiring their daughter and the foetal heart of twin two was okay. By 9.20, Julie was getting some contractions and was helped onto all fours in case it was a breech. Dad took his daughter and tucked her under his shirt. At 9.38, Julie got back onto the birthing stool to assist descent of head, pushing involuntarily. Andrea stood behind her and wrapped her arms round her to support her abdominal muscles while the other midwife checked the foetal heart rate.

'At 10.03, Julie was lying on her left side on the sofa and the foetal heart rate was increasing. Julie took some Caullophyllum 200 (homeopathic remedy). At 10.12 the head was visible, and at 10.13 twin two was born. The heart rate was strong and normal. The baby was received by the hospital midwife, dried and 'rubbed up'. Baby pinked up rapidly and was passed to Julie. Both parents were over the moon as they welcomed their son. We helped Julie to recline on the sofa, and at 10.18, both placentae were delivered. Julie lost about 450–500ml of blood [an average blood loss is around 150ml–200ml].

'I remained in attendance during the rest of the day while Julie continued to improve. By 4.30pm she was feeling very well and she had suckled both babies. I took down the intravenous drip that had been set up after the birth to replace fluid loss and to keep a vein open in the event of any further emergencies. Twin one, the girl, weighed 6lb 4oz/2.8kg and twin two, the boy, weighed 6lb 10oz/3kg. The uterus was very firm and Julie had afterpains. By 5.30pm, I felt that Julie's condition was now good and left the family in peace.'

[Julie did need a blood transfusion five days later because of the marked fall in blood pressure she had experienced during the birth. When I spoke to her she was still over the moon about her babies, describing the births as 'such easy births at home!']

Second-time-around mothers

'My husband said in wonder "it's a girl!" and Robbie Williams was singing "Angels" as she was passed to me…'

Caroline Watton, aged 39 and 10 months (she generously said I could call her 40), had her identical twin girls – Martha and Josie – after a requested induction at 39½ weeks. The twins shared one placenta, and she had a natural birth.

'I wanted to be induced at 38 weeks because I was so uncomfortable and had frankly had enough. The consultant at Chelsea & Westminster insisted I wait a week and booked me for induction on Monday 23 November when I was 39 weeks and two days.

'I rang the hospital on the Monday at 7am to check whether we could come in, but they told us they were too busy. I knew this might happen but Phil [Caroline's husband] and I had really psyched ourselves up for the birth, and we felt quite deflated. Rang again at midday as requested but still a no-go, so we went out to lunch and then to the cinema (still can't believe I managed to fit in one seat). Glad that I told family and friends that I wasn't being induced until Thursday…

'The next day I rang the hospital at 7am and with fingers crossed I was told we were on. Pretty excited and nervous en route to Chelsea & Westminster Hospital. Arrived around 9am and was taken straight through to the delivery unit and put on the monitor. Then at 10.30am our midwife broke my forewaters. I opted for gas and air during the process as it was pretty uncomfortable. Definitely now past the point of no return! Walked around for an hour to see if contractions started – they didn't.

'Back on the twin monitor, the heartbeats were steady at around 135. During late pregnancy and labour, I'd had three different midwives say pretty certainly that we were having boys – apparently boys tend to have a heartbeat range of 135 to 145 and girls above. An old wives' tale as it turned out.

'Jane, a very nice medical student, sat with us. We all read newspapers and tried to do a crossword. No contractions to speak of. At midday, they took a scan and both twins were head down.

'At 1.10pm, Nick the anaesthetist put the "mobile" epidural in – a little uncomfortable but soon forgotten and I definitely didn't want to be without one. A Syntocin drip is set up to try and start some contractions.

'The afternoon continued uneventfully – Phil, me and the medical student, plus various midwives popping in. I remained on the monitor and occasionally the line dipped dramatically – the first time this happened we pressed the emergency bell, but thankfully it was simply the belt slipping. After the initial scare, I learnt to reposition the belt and get the heartbeats back.

'At 6.30pm, I felt a little despondent after an internal examination revealed I was only 2cm dilated. It looked like a long night ahead.

'At 7pm, an internal pressure monitor was fitted (to me, not the babies) to allow them to 'up' the Syntocin to try and help speed things up. A television was brought in and Mel, a chatty New Zealand midwife, was now with us. We all watched a programme about weddings and had a good chat about children. Mel had a one-year-old boy – the only midwife I've had so far who has actually given birth!

'At 8pm, Phil was very keen to watch Liverpool versus Real Madrid – various people popped in, including Nick the anaesthetist, to see the match, not me! Score nil-nil (on pitch and in delivery room). As they were all absorbed by the match, I'd been swigging on the gas and air and starting to feel a bit woozy. Despite the epidural, I could feel some very strong contractions and hoped they would "up" the epidural as I wasn't enjoying this bit at all. My policy is 'why suffer when you don't need to?' and I've been very lucky with my previous two labours – epidurals for both resulting in straightforward deliveries, and not one stitch.

'At 10pm, I was 9cm dilated! Huge relief. I moved onto all fours and reluctantly parted company with the gas and air. Nick "upped" the epidural, which was very effective, and I started to look forward to the birth again. As I reached 10cm, the midwife speculated that we could deliver one prior to midnight and one after, which diverted my thoughts to separate birthday parties and boasts of being older by one day.

'Midnight: a new day – November 25. They wheeled the bed, with me still on all fours with drips attached, down the corridor and into the operating theatre. Lots of people are in there – Mel told me to ignore them all, dimmed the lights to 'romantic' level and tuned in the radio to some mellow music. An enthusiastic senior house officer tried to get me moved onto the operating table, but Mel told her firmly that I'd only move when and if it was necessary (with a thumbs up from the George Clooney-lookalike consultant).

'Still on all fours, and thankfully facing away from the audience, pushing commenced. At 1.15am, a little head appeared with eyes wide open, looked straight at the audience and then from side to side – one more push and we were there, what a relief!

"Is he okay?" I gasped. Phil says in wonder "It's a girl!" – and Robbie Williams is singing "Angels" as she is passed to me.

'Then the team became active. I'm was sitting up and hands were bearing down on my stomach to keep the position of twin two. Pushing recommenced – instead of exhaustion, adrenalin was high – the baby emerged arm-first and was pushed back inside and repositioned for the birth. At 1.46am, our second beautiful girl was born and there I was, the mother of identical twins.

'I remember very little about the placenta being delivered, so it must have been uneventful. All I remember was total elation – I cried tears of joy and relief at the safe arrival into the world of Martha Isabella and Josephine (Josie) Alice, who weighed in at 6lb 4oz/2.8kg and 5lb 8oz/2.5kg respectively.'

'At 41 weeks, my consultant greeted me with, "What are you doing here?"

Sarah Evans gave birth naturally to her non-identical girls, Lucy and Charlotte, at 41 weeks in St Thomas' Hospital in London. Having been induced with her first daughter, she didn't want to be induced with the twins.

'After the initial shock and excitement of finding out at my 12-week scan that we were expecting twins, my first visit to the obstetrician was rather deflating and negative. I was told to expect "double trouble" during the pregnancy – nausea, piles, varicose veins, indigestion and premature babies. I had been very sick during the first three months of my first pregnancy and was very sick again with my twin pregnancy, but not "doubly" so – not enough to suspect twins anyway (although I did say to both my mother and a very close friend the evening before the first scan, "I'll know tomorrow whether we're expecting twins" with no evidence but a sleepless night thinking about it and a general feeling. My maternal grandmother was a twin so maybe that fuelled the feeling but I had no such thoughts during my first pregnancy). The sickness persisted to about four months, and once my equilibrium was restored, I had a very healthy pregnancy with the only discomfort being that of rib ache and size at the end of the pregnancy.

'Everything I read or was told about expecting twins indicated that I was unlikely to be still pregnant after 38 weeks, so I was ready and waiting by 36 weeks, not daring to venture far. At 37 weeks, my mother's help, Christine, arrived so she would have a week or so to get to know Rosanna, then a very demanding 22-month-old. August slipped by (my due date was 27 August) but still no twinges. I was not expecting to be early because I had been induced with Rosanna at 42 weeks, but my consultant was increasingly surprised to see me every week. At 41 weeks, she greeted me with "What are you doing here?" When she examined me I was 2–3 cm dilated. However, as both the babies and I were absolutely fine, she listened as I explained that I did not want to be induced because Rosanna was very ill at the time with a virus and my first labour, following induction, had been a very long and difficult one.

'After 1 September, I decided that I really was ready, having held out until September, preferring my twins to be old for the school year. A stimulating aromatherapy massage on 2 September was unproductive and it was three days later when my waters broke at 12.30am on the birthday of my maternal grandmother (the twin). My first contraction was half an hour later and Lucy was born at 3.30am, weighing 6lb 2oz/2.8kg and Charlotte at 4am weighing 7lb 3oz/3.2kg. My husband was home in time for breakfast with Rosanna!

'The labour was excruciating as the contractions were so close together and intense from the outset, but it was mostly positive pain as things were moving so fast! Prior to examination, however, I was stuck on my back for what seemed an interminable age as the medical staff tried (unsuccessfully) to locate a twin monitor, and then to assess the babies' positions and monitor their heart-beats and the contractions. I was given gas and air, and at some point a Syntocin drip was inserted, but the details are all a bit hazy. By the time I had my initial examination, I was fully dilated and it was too late for an epidural.

'Lucy was delivered once I got the hang of pushing, and I held her briefly. But there was no time for cooing or putting to the breast as hands were immediately laid firmly on Charlotte to feel her position, and my feet were hoisted up into stirrups so that the doctors could break the waters of the second sac. The drip was then turned on or up to get the contractions going again as they had slowed down after Lucy's birth, and the midwife delivered Charlotte about 10 minutes later. I was able to breastfeed both babies soon after the birth. Fortunately, I had no stitches so was soon feeling fairly fit and normal – a very different story from Rosanna's birth.

'Undoubtedly a twin pregnancy and labour is more complicated that a singleton one, but I think it is important to be aware that, provided all is well, induction is not compulsory, even when over-due, and that it does not have to be routine to have an epidural.'

A section on sections

While a natural twin birth may be preferable in every respect, not everyone is going to be able to have one. Nor should there be any sense of failure or self-blame if the birth does not go according to plan. Of course, the most important thing in the world is that you are blessed with two healthy babies, and if you are blessed with two babies born by Caesarean section, then you may find that they are among the most peaceful babies on the planet. Don't ask me why that is, but it often seems to be the case.

Research reported in the *British Medical Journal* in October 2002 studied 4,500 twin births in Scotland over a five-year stretch. It concluded that because there was a greater risk of death to the second twin if born naturally, all twins should be delivered by Caesarean. While everybody agrees that safety is paramount, many midwives and obstetricians have contested the conclusions of the study and urged hospitals not to change their practice. If your doctor quotes this study when recommending a Caesarean, ask for a second opinion. If you want a natural birth, try to find a practitioner who is both committed to natural delivery and experienced. The benefits of natural over Caesarean are as much to do with the health of the mother as well as the babies. Fatalities during Caesarean section are estimated to be between 3 to 11 times higher than with vaginal delivery. A study in the *Journal of the American Medical Association* reported 1 to 2 maternal deaths per 1,000 operations and morbidity (non-fatal complications) at 8 to 10 times higher than with vaginal delivery.

However, for all the damning statistics, there are times when Caesareans are life-savers, such as during labour if there are signs of foetal distress or prolapsed cord (when the waters break, the baby's cord very occasionally comes down in front of their head). A section may need to be planned ahead of labour for medical reasons, such as placenta praevia (when the placenta lies partially or completely over the cervix) or abruption of the placenta (when the placenta begins to separate from the walls of the uterus). Other maternal problems include high blood pressure, diabetes, pre-eclampsia or if the babies are deemed not to be growing well. Sometimes, as in the case of Jo Pinkess (*below*), it may be recommended to you because of your existing history of Caesareans – and big babies.

Once the decision has been made for a Caesarean birth, you are prepared, or prepped, for surgery. Usually the consultant will go through procedures with you well in advance so you are properly informed. The mother's blood is drawn to be typed and cross-matched; an intravenous drip is inserted into her arm for administering fluids, medication or blood, and a catheter is inserted into her bladder. To monitor heartbeat and blood pressure, the mother will be fitted with a cuff and attached to a cardiac monitor.

Unless the pregnant woman has asked for a general anaesthetic, which is unusual these days, a spinal block or epidural will be given. There is the option of having a screen put up so the surgical side of delivery does not have to be witnessed. The father or birth partner will change into sterile clothing and that infamous green hat in preparation. Once the anaesthetic has taken effect, the birth begins.

'Both of my other deliveries had no complications and I healed up really well. Good Irish stock!'

Joanne Pinkess, 41, already had two children – Isabelle, 9, and Olivia, 6, when she fell pregnant with the twins. Both of her previous deliveries had been by Caesarean section – the first emergency, the second planned. At the birth of her twins, Caitlin weighed 8lb/3.6kg and Emily 7lb 5oz/3.3kg – a total weight of 15lb 5oz/6.9kg of baby.

'With the twins, I knew I wasn't even going to try for a natural birth. There is too much in the papers about the lack of midwives and too many people with stories of midwives not being there at the right time, or not having the level of experience to deliver twins – particularly to a 40-year-old woman who has already had two C-sections. Both of my other deliveries had no complications and I healed up really well. Good Irish stock! I didn't even find the not driving a bore [mothers who deliver by Caesarean are advised not to drive for six weeks] because I was so wiped out I didn't want to go anywhere. I do get quite anaemic, however, and I wasn't offered a blood transfusion with Isabelle and Olivia, only with the twins.

'I found out about the twins at my 13-week scan. At the time, I was more worried about the test for Down's syndrome. Five years earlier, when I was pregnant with Olivia, the test had given us a high chance (1 in 50) for my age of having a Down's syndrome baby. At the time, we decided to go ahead with the pregnancy without finding out for sure by having amniocentesis with its risk of miscarriage.

'So, five years on, I was very worried about that 13-week scan because I was now 40. When the sonographer turned to me and Andy and said, "Oh, I've got a bit of a shock for you," I immediately thought something was wrong with the baby. But Andy was looking at her face and could see she was smiling. "You have two in there." Andy was laughing and I was sobbing. People say, "Joanne, you should have known. Your mother has twin brothers, your sister has twins," but it had never even crossed my mind.

'I was a working woman. I didn't have time for twins. I see myself as an in-control kind of person, and it was the first time I felt really out of control. Andy thought it was so cool.

'Choosing your child's birthday is a really difficult thing to do when you plan a C-section. They get out their appointment book as if you are going to the dentist. It was terrible, really hard. You only have a degree of choice and I was set to be admitted at 39$^{1}/_{2}$ weeks, so we picked that date.

'It was only the two weeks before I had them that were tough. There was a lot of hanging about. On the day, you think that it's one of the most important moments of your life, and that you'll go in and everyone will cluck around you. So you roll in on your delivery day at 7.30am and nothing happens for 45 minutes. Slowly, the procedures start: filling out forms, putting on a gown, being processed. There's no-one coming over to you and saying, "Aren't you excited, Mrs Pinkess? This is your big moment," and I always think that's kind of a downer. So the nurse comes in to take your blood pressure and talks you through the procedure. As we were having an elected C-section, we had a briefing meeting the week before with a midwife who talked us through the whole process, and that is helpful.

'Then the consultant comes in and has a chat with you. More waiting around. I didn't go down into theatre until after 9am. I think I was the first of the day. We just strolled down, which was a strange feeling. Andy got into his scrubs and looked like something out of *ER*. He took three hits of whisky before he went in. We are not great people when it comes to all this, we are very squeamish.

'When you get in there, there are stacks of people – two midwives, two paediatricians, the consultant, the assistant surgeon, the anaesthetist, and then runners – about 10 altogether. So you get in there and they are all relaxed, and I find that they calm you a bit. It's just so routine for them, and that helps me to relax. And then they do the epidural, which is the bit I dread, but once that's in, that relaxes me, too.

'I bring my essential oils in, too: lavender and geranium because I like the smell. I put it on a piece of muslin and stick it on my chest, and everyone in the room is saying, "Wow, that smells wonderful, we should do this more often." I don't want to see what's going on so they put a screen up. And it is a strange sensation. As someone once said, it is as if someone is doing the dishes inside you. There is absolutely no pain though, and once you get used to that sensation, it isn't bad.

'So I strolled in at 9.30am and they were born at 10am and 10.01am. Once they are out, you don't care what is going on down below. A midwife said to me, "Are you sure you don't want them to bring the screen down so you can see them as they come out?" and I said no, because I have a tendency to faint. And I was worried that I was going to faint and miss it all. So I don't see the babies before they checked them and wrapped them, and then they put them on top of me. It is quite difficult because you are lying down, but I held them for a minute and handed them to Andy.

'He was just over the moon. The look on his face was just worth a million dollars because he was so excited. Within minutes I could tell their personality. We had picked the names and had to decide which one to give each twin. And I think it was about 20 minutes later that we named them. By then I could tell that Caitlin [weighing 8lb/3.6kg] was the feistier one and Emily [weighing 7lb 5oz/3.3kg] was more placid. They cried a little bit, which helps clear out their lungs. They were very calm when they came out.

'When the babies are out, they still have to sew you up. It takes longer to sew you up than to deliver the babies. It is probably about 15 minutes of putting you back together. It was a great atmosphere. Andy loved holding both of them and the midwives were taking pictures. The surgeon and the doctors joined in, but mainly it was the midwives who were clucking and cooing. But I was quite happy and they were a good team.

'I went to recovery about 11am. When they checked me at mid-day I was still bleeding too much. And then I had various doctors coming in and giving me internals, which was really invasive. The junior doctors didn't handle it very well. Then the consultant came in when they were about to do a transfusion. I didn't want to go back into theatre and I didn't want a transfusion. It's not just the HIV thing. I feel that if you can build up your own blood naturally, it's better than having someone else's.

'So she said, "I might be able to sort this but I need your help."
And she did a massive internal on me and it was horrible, but she
sorted me and I didn't have to go back in. But I was very anaemic
and my blood stores were not good.

'I was in hospital for five days, normal. I breastfed, but supplemented from the third day. For the first few days, you are very
sore and your mobility is quite restricted, and it is great that you
can ring the bell and someone takes up the baby and puts her on
your lap to feed. But the noise and food are awful in the hospital,
although Andy always brought in something special to keep me
well-fed.'

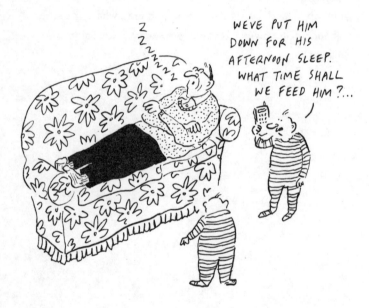

TEN

Congratulations! Congratulations! The Babies Are Here!

Unless you are an old hand at this motherhood business and need to get home to put the supper on, or unless you have an unholy fear of hospitals, you will have a lot to gain from your short stay in the maternity ward. You may have 'chosen' your hospital on the basis of the Starbucks coffee shop in close waddling distance, or because it was modern with lots of bright windows. Now that the babies are here, however, other, less superficial benefits are on hand.

Before the babies were born, all you cared about was that they would emerge into this world with all their fingers and toes, that the midwives would be kind, helpful and experienced, and the doctors paying attention. Now they are here, you can think of your hospital as a terrifically upmarket hotel, packed with helpful staff who KNOW WHAT THEY'RE DOING, available 24 hours a day at the press of a call button. If these are your first babies, don't rush to leave. You've paid your taxes; you deserve your bed as much as the next person, so make sure you wait until you are ready. If they ask whether you would like to go home today, and you don't feel you have mastered expressing milk on their automated breast pump, or want a fourth and fifth go at bathing the babies, don't go. Plead an inability to master feeding both twins at the same time if you must, but don't be pushed before you are ready. You will know when you can't bear another uncomfortable night in a single bed or the cries from somebody else's baby any longer. Then and only then are you ready for the comforts of your shag-pile carpet.

Most importantly, your stay in hospital is about gaining confidence in handling the babies. Like a really expensive hotel where you have to stop yourself taking the bath robes (because you've effectively paid for them), you want to take every bit of knowledge about looking after your babies with you when you leave. You (and your partner) may need to learn how to change nappies, wind a baby, give them a bath, clean their tummy button and – most importantly – breast-feed, before you are ready to leave. You probably feel disbelieving that anybody would let you leave without some sort of parental Girl-Guide certificate anyway.

Hospital food

The most fully-equipped, fully-staffed hotel in the world also has the worst food on the planet. I say this now because, at some stage after the babies are born, you are going to feel ravenously hungry, with no-one around to offer you so much as a snack. Be prepared (because even if they had, you wouldn't want to eat it). Ask your partner, mother, mother-in-law, best friend, nosy neighbour – anyone who wants to come in and visit – to pick up a picnic on the way. Marks and Spencer would be nice, but a few choice things from Sainsbury's or Tesco's deli will do just as well. Basket of fruit, tin of American muffins and cookies, anything foodie-orientated will be gobbled up (by your visitors as well as you). What nobody has told you yet is that when you breastfeed twins you will become so ravenously hungry that you will be tearing whole loaves in half.

Early bonding

Depending on how the birth went, you might find that bonding with two babies is not an instant thing. If you are recovering from a C-section, you may be wiped out, anaemic and horrified at the prospect of looking after anyone at that moment, unless it is poor prodded you. If you are nursing stitches, as well as two babies, you might feel overwhelmed by the physical enormity of what has just happened. This is utterly normal. It is universally acknowledged that it is a slower process bonding with twins anyway, not least because when you look lovingly at one, the other is squealing for attention.

What is less well known is how differently you may feel towards the two babies at the beginning. Even mothers of identical twins that are born with different birth weights report this. It may be that the heavier identical twin, who sleeps better and is less fussy on the breast, quickly becomes your favourite. Or, if you have boy/girl twins, the longed-for boy, or girl, is the one you choose to nuzzle up with when they both wake at the same time. These feelings are not unusual. They are to do with everything from your own earliest child-hood experiences to a cocktail of hormones spinning around your system, and things will eventually settle down. By the time your twins both reach a year, the idea of favourites will be laughable. You will favour the twin who is not clinging to your leg, throwing his broccoli on the floor and pulling down the Christmas tree. The next day you will favour the other twin who is not clinging to your leg, throwing the broccoli...

In the meantime, there is no point feeling any guilt around the matter. One of the best ways of avoiding feeling guilty is to air your preferences or unasked-for feelings to a midwife or trusted friend. Just the act of saying what you feel usually redresses the balance anyway, and you will find yourself com-pensating at the next feed by spending more time with the other baby.

Other areas of guilt that are delivered with the placenta may concern the birth itself. If the birth did not go according to plan, you may have irrational feelings of failure, or if the babies need to spend some time in the neo-natal unit, you may have feelings of guilt about your second glass of wine in the first trimester. Again, this is more a psychological limber-ing up for the responsibility of motherhood. Every mother on the planet harbours such thoughts, and don't let them be swept aside by concerned partners. Find someone to talk to about it who understands. Other mothers of twins or girl-friends with more than one child are best. And if you start a blubbing chain reaction in your triumphant post-natal NCT class, the others will thank you for it later.

Bonding with dada

Hospitals are also good places to enlist the help of the professionals to train your partner. It will be much better that a nurse shows him how to change a nappy properly than you. Connive with the midwives in your plans. Midwives and nurses know that it is just as much part of their jobs to include fathers in the post-natal care, so persist in finding someone who will help. AT NO POINT SHOULD YOU FEEL YOU ARE WASTING PROFESSIONAL TIME. You will be checking out of this expensive hotel very shortly, so make sure you use all the facilities while you are there. You have just become the most important and valued member of society – a mother. You deserve every ounce of help that the state can offer you (as well as the TWO bounty bags that the private sector is offering). Daddy getting experience in bathing his babies in the jovial atmosphere of the hospital nursery will feel like a lot more fun than panicking alongside you at home.

Should you worry for one second that the nurses or midwives seem too busy with other more urgent and important work, bear in mind the words of my friend, a nurse, Claire. Having worked on all the hospital wards, she let me into the secret that despite the air of busyness that a maternity ward gives off, the nurses are actually nowhere near as run off their feet as in other wards, where they are caring for genuinely sick people, wholly dependent on nurses for their care. So, if the nurses seem to be dashing past you, or too busy to answer your call, press again. They are probably only rushing to put the kettle on and open the newest donated box of Roses chocolates.

Most fathers of twins are immediately better at caring for their babies than fathers of singletons anyway. They have to be, because someone has to hold one baby while the other is being attended to. Encourage his involvement as much as possible. Tell him how he looks like a natural, even when he is holding your darling little newborn in a slightly uncomfortable way, and you're dying to rush up to him and pull the poor child from his arms. Just smile through those gritted teeth and tell him HOW MUCH THE BABY LOOKS LIKE HIM. I don't know why this always works with fathers, but it does. Must be some genetic thing with Undisputed Paternity.

What you want is a father who is territorial and puffed up with pride over your twins, not one who feels alienated and a bit spare. So, even in those first few days when you don't feel like you have enough time to go to the loo, practise including your partner every moment you are together. It will pay off in the long run, I promise.

Bonding with other siblings

When pregnant with the twins, I was fixated about how my three-year-old would react to his whole world being overturned overnight by the arrival of two little terrorists (invading the house, making it look like a bomb has hit it, waking you up at all times of the night). I called Jane Denton, the head of the Multiple Births Foundation, and she suggested two little tricks, both of which worked well for me.

The first was that the babies bought a present for my eldest son, something special that he would associate with their arrival. At the time, Humphrey was obsessed with Lego and Action Man, so Michael 'bought' him Action Man Polar Bike Explorer and Millie 'bought him' a huge box of Lego. Two years later, he still reminds me that these presents came from 'my twins'.

The other suggestion was to allow Humphrey to choose two special teddies for the twins that would become their comforters as time went by. As the teddies were always present in their Moses basket or cots, it gave my son a small stake in the fuss made around the babies.

Another tip picked up from the school gate was to ask people who came to visit to bring a present for Humphrey, rather than for the babies. This made every visit an event. Just by asking people to remember him made others more aware of his importance as new big brother, and more sensitive to barging past him to coo over the babies.

Finally, I found stopping people at the door and asking if Humphrey could show the visitor where 'his twins' were, also helped him feel included. He would then lead the person to the Moses basket, as though wholly responsible for producing this spectacle, and I'd stand back to let him take all the credit for how cute they were.

Of course, your time and attention is far more valuable than any number of Tonka toys that are heaped upon other siblings around the birth of the twins. One friend and mother of three was given some advice by a nurse in the hospital before being released back into the world. 'If you can spend one hour a day with each child, you will never find that they suffer from sibling rivalry.' She did, and they don't. I have never met three more well-adjusted teenagers, happy to be in each other's company and boasting of each other's qualities. I, personally, have never achieved this goal, but giving each child some special time in the day by, say, staggering bed-times, also works. As Adele Faber and Elaine Mazlish note in their book *Siblings Without Rivalry*: 'Where does it all begin? The experts in the field seem to agree that at the root of sib-ling jealousy is each child's deep desire for the exclusive love of his parents.' If you can offer them their own exclusive time with you, when they are not competing for attention with anyone or anything else, then you could save yourself a lot of fighting in the future.

The grand thing about grandparents

Grandparents are a godsend when you have babies. Even if you are still in a fight with your father for refusing to top up your student loan, or still angry with your mother for ruin-ing your favourite sweater (or divorcing your father), the arrival of your children is the right time to change all that. Now the pendulum has swung in their favour. Before chil-dren, a day visiting your parents might not have been top of your list, but now the prospect of some safe and loving arms in which to hand over a baby is more appealing than a week-end at the Ritz.

What is more, there is no greater bond than that of a grandparent and a grandchild (all that love and genetic heritage, with none of the responsibility) and it should be encouraged on every level. Grandparents are among the few people who really, really care if little Timmy is having a hard time sleeping through the night as he cuts his first teeth. They will listen patiently as you use them to work out whether baby is still hungry and thirsty after taking two ounces at his last feed and sleeping for five minutes. Although at times it may be irritating to get the fifth call of the day about their progress, you must grin and bear it. The rewards shall be reaped, not in heaven, but here on earth when baby-sitting, or a weekend away, beckons. Grandparents of twins, unless they are too frail or uninterested, should be flattered, cajoled and spoilt with every handprint picture to get them on board from day one.

If you are lucky enough to have two sets of grandparents who are equally able and willing to fawn on their offspring's offspring, they should be played off against each other ruthlessly to encourage a competitive spirit. 'Gosh! How lovely you are going off on your booze cruise to France. The other Granny is coming up specially to see the children to take them on a Santa spectacular.' This kind of shameless name-dropping means that the next phone call will be Granny offering you a night off, promising to come armed with French champagne and to stuff Christmas stockings.

If you are shocked by such behaviour, settle for including the grandparents as much as possible in the early days, weeks and years with the children. It will be hard for you at times, being elbowed out of the way at the door so Granny can bestow on your darlings strictly forbidden sweeties before lunchtime. But try and enjoy it. Even better, use the time to announce that you are going for a swim – grannies prefer to be in charge for small amounts of time so that they can really break the rules.

Equally hard is when you see that you are no longer Daddy's little girl, but that Grandpa has got eyes only for the next generation of bewitching babes. Remember, he had to go through losing you to your partner a while ago, and now you are having to experience the same kind of loss. Arrival of new babies always entails a shift in the power balance of a family. Things will settle down again soon enough, and you will get used to being a yummy mummy instead.

Everything changes when you have children. New and unexpected bonds and relationships are formed. It is in your interest to smooth over the running of this complicated clock and keep the wheels oiled with little photographs to the grandparents and mementos to cousins. One day, you will be able to call them up and say 'Mum, I need a night off.' And then they will come running.

And who cares about me?

Another reason for staying a reasonable length of time in hospital is because this is where the lovely nurses will also be looking after *you*, as well as helping you to care for your babies. When I had my first child, my elderly neighbour reminisced about her early days of motherhood with her only son. She told me that in her day, mothers were cosseted in the local cottage hospital for two whole weeks. Every day they would be made to lie on their stomachs in order to deflate the tummy(!), and were pampered and cooked for, while a team of prim nurses took the babies away at night to let the mothers sleep. What bliss. And we call our short stay in hospital 'progress'.

Certain aspects of a twin pregnancy may mean recovery is a little slower. 'Twin skin' – the result of your stomach being stretched that bit further by two babies – means that it can take a little longer for your uterus to go down. The afterpains of your uterus contracting, felt particularly when breastfeeding, can either feel painful or – some lucky mothers report – like post-coital vibrations. Let's hope for your sake it's the latter.

I won't bother to be a hypocrite and espouse the value of post-natal exercises, as the only exercise I ever took in those early days was folding back the duvet to dive in fully clothed. However, if you are concerned about regaining your figure as soon as possible, take advantage of the hotel, sorry hospital, facilities to ask whether there is a resident physiotherapist or a midwife specializing in this area who might take time to go through an exercise programme with you. Once again, it is all part of your post-natal care, so you are quite within your rights to ask for it. Should you ever worry that you are 'making a fuss', console yourself with the thought that you will probably never see these nurses again. So if they do have to explain for the third time a simple latching-on procedure that they showed you yesterday, don't feel embarrassed. It is what they are there for.

Postpartum dementia and primary maternal preoccupation

These phrases, invented by our American friends, neatly sum up the 'milk for brains' state that creeps in shortly after birth. It is important to acknowledge that everyone, even captains of industry and the chairwoman of Coca Cola, suffers from it. It is caused by lack of sleep, an acute sense that only by focusing your attention on the babies will they thrive, adjustment to the huge change of becoming a mother, and the hormone oxytocin that courses through your veins after birth and during breastfeeding.

Postpartum dementia means that not only will you forget to have any food ready for your partner at the end of the day, you will forget that you even have a partner. And as for organizing to pick up his dry-cleaning or phone the plumber, you will swear he never mentioned it. Anticipating postpartum dementia means that if you can enlist someone else – doula, mother, girlfriend – to do some of the practical tasks, such as shopping, ironing and cleaning, then do. Shout 'Help!' Give them a spare set of keys, because no doubt you have lost your own along with your handbag sometime last week.

Another phrase that should be memorized (for the few seconds you can memorize anything now you are a mother) is Primary Maternal Preoccupation. This means that when your best friend is telling you her boyfriend has just left her for a gay lover, you will be interrupting her to ask whether she thinks the baby is too warm in his hooded top. Primary Maternal Preoccupation is nature's way of making you ignore the mess under the sink in favour of the transparent blueness of your babies' eyes. News and politics on the television will wash over you as if being beamed from another planet, while a Pampers advert with itchycoo babies on it will have you sobbing into your Kleenex. It is nature's way of preparing you for a new life. The world as you knew it before you had babies is different to the one you now inhabit. Your new world is infinitely richer, and more full of feelings, filled with all the wonder and vulnerability of human existence. Now you are a mother, enjoy it.

The dreaded 'D' word

Without wanting to play down the seriousness of a bout of full-blown postnatal depression (PND), often triggered by a chemical reaction to birth, I would like to say a short word about PND. Sue, a friend, healer and stress-management counsellor, believes that most mothers suffer from a touch of depression at some stage after their babies arrive. It is simply a reaction to the enormous physical, emotional and mental change they have just undergone, as well as the act of labour. That means that if you are feeling down, it is entirely understandable.

During my twin pregnancy, I had a mild period of depression early on when the joyous news of my twins brought with it the flip side of the coin – lack of freedom. Here I was, pregnant, delighted with the prospect of my expanded family but already mourning my past life with the relatively carefree existence of just one child. After the twins arrived, I was on such a high from the birth for months and months that the night feeds, crying and lack of sleep didn't bring on the baby blues as expected. However, just after their first birthday, tendrils of depression began to take root as I became irrationally obsessed with them growing up. Instead of wishing away their tiny lives, like many mothers do in the hope that children will get easier, I folded away every babygro that no longer fitted into the drawer with a nagging sense of unfairness. I didn't want my babies to grow up, I wanted them to stay the same, and I had this strange sense of time passing with me looking on helplessly.

Now this would never be classified as postnatal depression in a medical sense, but my friend Sue spotted it in my behaviour and put her finger on it. 'I think you've had a little bit of postnatal depression, my dear,' she said. Just by the act of labelling it, she helped it to pass, and sure enough it melted away as gently as it had arrived. The same weekend I was back at the make-up counter, wanting to buy a new outfit.

Your little bit of PND may come in a milder or stronger form, but there is nothing to fear from it. It may come in the form of compulsive behaviour – checking and rechecking the bottles to see whether they are sterilized; it may come in the form of an unsettling desire to want to avoid the babies (this is nothing to do with not loving them). It may centre around disappointment about the birth, or feelings of inadequacy and not being able to cope. It might be to do with your loss of identity, or fear of being alone, or feeling physically low, or waking nightmares about disasters happening to the babies. It may take the form of you finding no interest in previously enjoyable activities, and worrying that you will always feel like this.

The good news is that you won't. Everything, even the most difficult baby stage, will pass. The best advice is to try not to take it out on your partner because he is the nearest person to hand. He got you into this mess, you think. He is the babies' father, so why can't he do a full night of feeding? Remember that he, too, is adjusting to his new life, and he has even less access to any support than you do. He may even feel jealous of the new arrivals (yes, this does happen) because his partner has just fallen in love with two new human beings. Or been kidnapped by two squalling terrorists.

So, if you find yourself rowing, resist. Go dump on someone else instead – a trained counsellor, therapist, doctor, best friend, NCT co-ordinator, mother, midwife, health visitor – anyone but your partner. It is perfectly normal to find motherhood a challenge. If you have twins, you deserve everyone's sympathy and attention, so never worry about 'wasting someone's time'. If most mothers have some form of PND, whether they are aware of it or not, you are not alone. Sharing your feelings might help others to articulate their own. There. That's the Oprah bit over and done with.

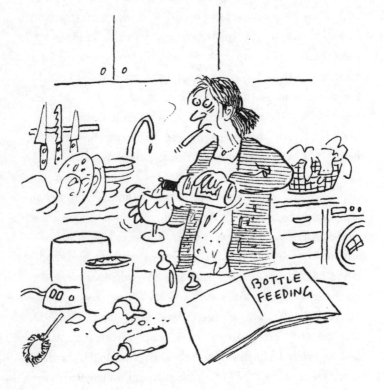

ELEVEN

The Gentlewomanly Art of Breastfeeding Twins

Ahhh, breastfeeding. It sounds so simple, doesn't it? You put a baby to the breast and they have ready-made food flowing with antibodies at just the right temperature. Think Jerry Hall naked with baby, think Madonna and Child. Nature is such a clever thing. So, why then is breastfeeding a huge hand-grenade of a topic associated with pain and guilt and feelings of inadequacy from those that can't or choose not to?

Well, I'm afraid it's all part of being a mother, with a good dose of our rotten-to-mother culture thrown in. The modern world puts on a pedestal skinny models and the achieving woman back at her desk (and then whispers over the photo-copier about anorexia and neglected children). Breastfeeding is still taboo as an outdoor spectacle, although brave mothers do still do it, and it is not an easy skill to learn. In fact, a mother who has decided to breastfeed her twins needs a lot of support, both from her partner – because she will spend a fair amount of time pinned to the sofa waving instructions, 'Sorry, I can't move, I'm feeding the babies' – and from a kindly granny figure (nurse, midwife, health visitor, breast-feeding counsellor). Everyone around you needs to will you to succeed in the early days, otherwise you may not.

The good news is that you'd be surprised at how many people out there genuinely do want you to succeed. A quick glance at the number of websites available for breastfeeding mothers (www.breastfeed.com and www.lalecheleague.org for starters) will give you some indication of how passionate the breastfeeding clan is. There are a lot of people who are keen to give you information to help you prepare and join their happy throng. Take advantage of it before or after the babies arrive. You will be welcomed with open arms into their ample bosoms.

The very best place to get it going, particularly if you are a first-time mother, is in hospital. Sarah Evans, who had successfully breastfed her first daughter until pregnant with her twins, upgraded to an NHS private room after her twin birth, and enjoyed the benefits of pressing a bell every time she needed help to latch both babies on. This is guaranteed in the private sector, but not so in a normal maternity ward, where you may have to shout loudly to get attention.

Nevertheless, those early days are extremely important and you have the excuse of needing help with one twin while the other latches on to get extra help in the hospital. **Heather Neil, an NCT breastfeeding counsellor and tutor, reckons that it is more than twice as difficult for a twin mother to breastfeed than a singleton mother.**

Breast is best

For twins, you may need a little more mental preparation than most, starting with a cast-iron belief that breast is best, and no-one will persuade you otherwise. Like any skill, breastfeeding has to be learnt, and it helps if you love it and want to get better at it. Without that fundamental belief that this is something you really want to do for the sake of your babies (and because there are lots of benefits for you), then the road to breastfeeding success will be a rocky one. Whatever you do – breastfeed, bottle-feed, mix-feed – promise me one thing: you won't beat yourself up about it if things don't work out as you planned. **Nobody ever tells you that there is an element of luck in breastfeeding.**

For all this effort, mothers of twins do get the immense satisfaction of knowing that they are giving their babies the very best start in life, protecting them against infection and allergies, as well as helping their own body get back to normal (breastfeeding helps the uterus to contract back to its original size). There is also the small matter of this wonderful drug called oxytocin, produced naturally by the body when breastfeeding. Oxytocin turns you from a stressed-out harpie into a smiling Mona Lisa. As your let-down reflex happens, and the babies start to suckle happily, this amazing feeling of calmness and relaxation kicks in. Nothing much matters at that moment, except your thriving babies and you. Oxytocin should be bottled and sold to harried husbands commuting home from work. They could swig on it before entering the house and slipping on the post still in the hallway.

Finally, there is one more benefit to breastfeeding your twins that can never be over-emphasized: you can eat up to 4,000 calories a day. So say hello to guilt-free Kettle Chips.

Babies come first

Breastfeeding is also a lifestyle decision. It is not something that can be slotted in to routines, an early return to work, a determination to get the baby to sleep through from day one or a desire to lose weight quickly (although you do lose weight breastfeeding, it just takes a little time). You are not supposed to diet when breastfeeding, so there is no question of dashing to the gym to return to your pre-pregnancy shape.

Breastfeeding is about giving yourself up to the babies and new motherhood, especially for the first few months when you and the babies are learning how to do it. Until you have mastered it, there will be crisis moments, usually at 3am, when you think about jacking it all in for a bottle of formula. (It's like an alcoholic's worst nightmare: the bottles are always there, glinting away in the cupboard, bought by a 'kindly' friend. And you know that if you take them, it might be the road to ruin.) But hang on to only one thought throughout all the sore nipples and painful latches in those early days: **breastfeeding suddenly becomes much easier after three months.** It is the magic time, when a lot of people ironically stop, when the baby can feed in a few minutes and you can wander around the house, barely noticing that you have a child swinging happily from your boob. Three months is all it takes. Put the date in your diary for when you are feeling desperate.

I comforted a best friend, a successful film business type, as she sobbed on my shoulder about failing as a mother. She had just returned from her first month's checkup and her son had not put on any weight for the third week running. She was tired, stressed out, and wasn't producing enough milk. It happens. By the second baby she was ready to admit that she 'hated breastfeeding and couldn't wait to give it up'. As a well-educated, middle-class mother, she knew it was best for the babies to be fed by breast, but her heart was never in it. For her, it was just another demand on her body.

Breast and bottle

The decision to mix bottle and breast is not a simple one because once you start introducing bottles, your milk supply dwindles. In our twins club survey, half of the mothers who introduced mixed feeding at birth or within the first week had given up by six weeks. The figures nationally show an even more dramatic drop. The Infant Feeding Survey 2000 compiled by the Department of Health showed that 40 per cent of breastfeeding mothers whose babies had been given a bottle while in hospital had stopped breastfeeding altogether by two weeks. Compare that to 13 per cent of breastfeeding mothers whose babies had not been given a bottle. So if you want the breastfeeding to work, the commitment has to be there from day one.

However, once you and baby have got the hang of it, there is no reason why you can't cheat a little, especially at the end of the day when your milk supply is down from tiredness and dehydration. At this early evening feed, **typically around 6pm, many mothers introduce a one-off bottle of formula for the twins**. It has many benefits. It allows a partner returning from work to give the feed, and therefore bond a little with their babies. It allows you to prepare a good meal to get your energy supply up for the evening ahead, and it gives you a few hours to rest, have a bath and other forgotten pleasures. Miranda Whiteley, who breastfed her twin boys until they were seven months, says 'I wouldn't have continued breastfeeding if I hadn't had someone else around and if we hadn't used formula at the crucial early evening feed and occasionally in the night.'

It is also worth alerting you ahead to the famed **six-week growth spurt.** Megan Landon, who breastfed her identical twin boys until they were 22 months old, and exclusively on breast milk until they were eight months old, described the six-week growth spurt as 'one of the only times in my whole baby days when I was reduced to tears'. It is the time when many fall to the formula. Megan also maintains that waking the other twin up to feed, rather than demand feeding, is the ONLY way to breastfeed twins.

Every little helps

Out of 50 mothers who responded to our local twins club survey, every single one of them had tried breastfeeding and lasted for a minimum of a couple of weeks. And even if you only give your newborns the colostrum – a straw-coloured fluid rich in vitamin K, proteins and antibodies that is produced in the first few days before your milk comes in – then you are giving them instant protection against gastroenteritis and other nasty bacteria. As the NCT handbook says: 'There are sound reasons for giving your baby a few days of breast milk, even if you would prefer not to breastfeed.'

If you can make it to around three months, the time when your twins will turn from fragile newborns into bouncing babies, then you will reach the critical stage when breastfeeding becomes easier. NCT breastfeeding counsellor Heather Neil explains that this is the time when most babies become much quicker at draining a breast, and can take their feed in as little as five or six minutes (a lot quicker than any baby can down a bottle).

But, as every twin mother and lactation consultant will agree, it is often getting to that three-month stage that is the hardest part. Breastfeeding is as much about the baby as it is about the mother, and a twin mother nursing two babies is a living example of how one baby can be fussy and difficult to feed while another is relatively easy. All can learn; some are just more willing pupils than others.

There is a learning curve for you, too. Once you have got them both latched on and are ready to go, you have no hands to turn a newspaper, reach for a glass of water or the remote control. Twin breastfeeders have to learn to become experts in having long telephone conversations with the mobile in the crook of their neck while kicking the dog out of the way of the TV with their feet.

Feeding apart

This debate will be raging long after you have put your twins through university. There are, of course, benefits to feeding together and apart, but at the end of the day it comes down to different styles. Mothers like Sarah Evans, 34, who fed her two separately, was blessed with two good feeders who didn't fuss for hours at the breast and therefore made the whole process pleasurable. Sarah designated each of the twins one of her breasts, and fed them on demand for four months exclusively. After four months, when bottles and other foods were introduced, she still carried on giving the odd feed to her girls up until they were eight months old.

Gaia Pollini, meanwhile, preferred to feed her boy twins separately for the first three months while they were both getting the hang of it, and then together after that when suddenly it all became easier. Now, at a year old, they still prefer a top-up from Mum to their Italian meatballs.

The benefits of nursing the twins separately are obvious. It allows you special time with each one, as well as giving you a free hand with which to eat your snacks or wave the flash cards at twin two. It also stops you feeling like the Bearded Lady if anyone should drop in for a cup of tea and suddenly be faced by a full frontal. Feeding sequentially is the ONLY way of nursing your twins when out and about.

Unless you want to strip to the waist and audition for Page Three.

Feeding together

Some twins actually feed better together. Call it a twin thing, or that the babies prefer the closeness of Mum and their womb-mate. The benefit for the mother is speed. If you have both feeding together then the feed takes as long (in theory) as a single baby. In practice, one baby may fall asleep halfway through, while the other feeds more quickly. Or one may need winding over your shoulder halfway through, while the other has yet to finish.

The favourite feeding position for both at the same time is called, attractively, the Double Football Hold (take a photograph of yourself doing it and you will know why). To do it, you rest both babies on a cushion, holding their heads like two melons up to your breasts. Once you become professional at this – and everyone will have a preference for which cushions, edge of the sofa, one-handed grip on the babygro that they use – you can even take both hands away. Look Mom! No hands!

One of the less-talked about advantages of the Double Football Hold is that it can transform two noisy babies into two quiet ones, within seconds. My three-year-old Humphrey would often ask in the early days, 'Mummy, would you feed the babies now please? I want to watch my video.'

What about feeding one and not the other?

Of course this is possible, and with one extremely fussy little girl baby and one placid bouncing boy baby, I am ashamed to admit that I did do this for a while. Of course, I fully expect to pay my daughter's therapy bills when she tells this to her shrink in years to come. If you can take the guilt, it is one way of keeping the feeding going in the hope that the other baby may take to it later on. If this happens to you, this is the stage to call in a lactation consultant (*see addresses below*) or visit a successful breastfeeding mother in your twins club (most have a designated breastfeeding support person) to sit and chat through some problems. A lactation consultant may watch you feed the baby and notice some physical or positioning problem that is making it harder. For example, in my case, the lactation consultant noticed that my little girl had a high palate, which made latching on that much more difficult.

Going back to work

Although breastfeeding handbooks might suggest that you blithely pop into the ladies at work with your breast pump and emerge triumphant with a pint in each hand, most of us know that the reality is somewhat different. Even if you do have a fridge at work, labelling your milk 'Baby Michael' and 'Baby Millie' might not go down well with the boys in the post room (and let's hope it's never used at teatime by mistake). Megan Landon, who went back to work when her twins were seven months, did manage to overcome obstacles to keep the feeding going. She used an Avent hand pump to express her milk in the day, tried to organize meetings so that she wasn't stuck somewhere without a room to do it, and brought in a cool bag to transfer the milk from the fridge to home. When she walked through the door in the evening she was 'wrestled to the ground' by her two boys who were keen to climb onto Mummy's lap and get their just desserts. Reason enough to keep going.

If you can keep the feeding going when you get home, you may find that doing a feed once in the night is something that helps you unwind. I know one mother (a twin herself) who found feeding her son at night during her full-time job gave her this wonderful, special time with her baby (now two, and still getting it), as well as assuaging some of the guilt from leaving him for the workplace.

Feeding stuff

Breast pumps

An electric breast pump with double adaptor so that both breasts can be milked at once is the Rolls Royce of gadgets to have in the house. The battery ones are a little noisy for my taste, although I know plenty of mothers who express only occasionally and get on very well with them. As my first child was a cleft baby who could only be fed with expressed milk,

I have always used Expressions Breastfeeding (01538 386650) who rent Medela Lactina Electric double breast pumps at £42 for the first 10 days, and £18 per month thereafter (including delivery and all the bits). An unwieldy, car battery-sized thing, it is fantastically quiet and efficient, but extremely unsexy. Otherwise check the parenting mags for the hottest new pump.

V-shaped cushion

This cushion is a potential New Best Friend that lifts your babies' head up to the right level for the breasts. It always comes out as the top buy in every twins club survey, and can be found in all John Lewis department stores. Smart versions can be found with a Velcro strap that wraps around the back, adding a little extra support for posture.

Bottles

If you want to mix-feed, and don't want your babies to become 'nipple confused' or prefer the bottles to the breast, the latex-teated Playtex Feeding systems are recommended by lactation consultants. They also work for mainly breastfed babies who need topping up. The Playtex systems have these plastic bag inserts that collapse as the milk is drunk and therefore reduce the amount of air, and wind, that the baby gets. The bags are thrown away afterwards, so there is no need to sterilize the bottles, although the teats have to be boiled or steamed. Playtex systems are available from most independent small chemists.

If you plan to mix-feed later, **introduce a bottle early on with a little bit of cooled boiled water**, just to acquaint the babies with the idea of something foreign that also can be sucked for fluid. It makes the transition a lot easier should you decide to change over to bottles later.

Sterilizers

These get better and better every year, so it is a perfect excuse to buy another copy of *Practical Parenting* magazine or *You and Your Baby* to coo over other people's perfectly turned-out infants. Make sure you buy one that takes the maximum number of bottles.

Breastfeeding books

If you plan to nurse, it is a good idea to have a proper doorstopper of a breastfeeding book to keep the door open as you shout instructions to your partner downstairs. The best bibles, recommended by breastfeeding twin mothers, are: *Bestfeeding: Getting Breastfeeding Right for You,* Celestial Arts, May 2000; *Mothering Multiples: Breastfeeding and Caring for Twins or More!* by Karen Gromada, La Leche League International, 1999 (currently unavailable in UK, but both can be purchased from Amazon.com).

Common breastfeeding myths

Myth 1: Breastfeeding is cheaper

I am sorry to go out on a limb, but the amount of shopping and eating that was needed to sustain my rapacious appetite during my breastfeeding weeks as a twin mother discounted any savings on formula milk. A breastfeeding twin mother keeping up her calorie intake to nurture three people has to think carefully about what she eats and when. Unless you live on an organic farm, this is expensive in the days of weekly shops in Sainsbury's and Tesco's.

Myth 2: Breastfeeding helps mothers regain their figures

Breastfeeding helps mothers regain their figures *eventually* would be more honest. As well as that wonderful full breast-feeding buxom bosom, the body is not keen to get rid of any fat stores until absolutely necessary when producing milk. Mothers who try and lose weight while breastfeeding report, quite simply, that they can't. Sure, the weight drops off slowly as the months go on, but dieting is out of the question.

Myth 3: Breastfeeding saves time

Mmmmm. Tricky one this. Breastfeeding is something that only a mother can do. Husbands, partners, doulas and cleaning ladies can sterilize bottles and make up feeds for the whole day ahead. They can also give the babies a bottle. So breastfeeding saves time for husbands, partners, doulas and cleaning ladies, might be more accurate.

Myth 4: Breastfeeding is nature's contraceptive

Only because sex while breastfeeding in the early days feels like yet another demand on your body, this time wreaked by a large hairy male rather than an exquisite soft-skinned newborn. Plus, unless you hop from the nursery to the double bed, your boobs are always engorged or engorging, and this is painful stuff. I can count at least two friends who have taken the myth of breastfeeding equals contraception to heart, and expanded their family in the process. While breastfeeding reduces the incidence of ovulation, and many women may not ovulate while they are lactating, this is not the case for every woman, particularly fertile two-egg twin mums.

Breastfeeding benefits

Breastfeeding is one of life's most sensuous experiences. The very rightness of a tiny baby nuzzling into your chest and the utter sense of relaxation that follows after let-down, when you feel that no other job in the world is as important as this, is a truly wonderful aspect of motherhood. Some women hide from their partners quite how much they enjoy the feeling, particularly when sex is often the last thing on their mind. Some mothers even whisper about uterine contractions during breastfeeding akin to post-coital vibrations. Keep this quiet, too.

Breastfeeding is wonderful for bonding. Once your twins are up and running around, you will feel more like a waitress fetching and carrying than a mother. Breastfeeding your babies is a precious time spent together that very soon will seem a long way away. These are moments when you can watch your baby and enjoy his or her very differentness from the other. Forget television – playing with your baby's fingers or rearranging a loose curl is the most valuable pastime in the world.

Breastfeeding is a great excuse for sitting down a lot. Getting horizontal, or failing that, sitting down, will become your greatest fantasy as you enter new motherhood. As the old joke goes, 'What does every mother want in bed?' Answer: 'Eight hours.' When you are breastfeeding, you are forced to sit down and do nothing but feed the babies (and how much more important a job can you get than that?). So others have to do all the boring drudgery such as stacking dishwashers.

Breastfeeding can always get you out of a tight squeeze. Whether it's a good reason to leave a party early or the best excuse to pull over in a traffic jam, if you are breastfeeding you are never going to feel that cold pang of fear that very shortly you are going to have a caterwauling that only food can stop. If you are breastfeeding, you are never going to be caught short without a bottle. No small matter with twins.

Breastfeeding is better for the babies. The amazing thing about our bodies is that breast milk does actually change to meet the nutritional needs of the babies. So the milk you produce in the first three months is different to the milk you produce later on. How does our body know that? How can it be so clever?

Useful telephone numbers

I know these are supposed to be given at the end of the book, but you need every bit of extra help (like not wading through irrelevant addresses) to get this breastfeeding thing cracked. Fortunately, there are many people, mostly mothers and volunteers, out there to help you at any time of day or night who really do care that you make it work. Here are a few of their numbers.

The National Childbirth Trust (NCT) Breastfeeding support line (0870 444 8708)

The line is run by trained volunteers who will visit you at home, if possible, if you need special help. The NCT line has a register of breastfeeding mothers and can put you in touch with another twin mother to chat through any particular difficulties.

Twins and Multiple Births Association (TAMBA: 0870 770 3305)

TAMBA has a good booklet called *Breastfeeding Twins, Triplets and More* that shows all the different positions in which you can attempt to feed your twins. Also, perhaps more helpfully once you have started feeding, they have a new video showing mothers breastfeeding their twins and demonstrating how to do it no-handed. Also their **Twinline** (0870 770 3303), manned by parents on weekdays between 7pm and 11pm, weekends 10am to 11pm, is not specifically set up to support breastfeeding but can help put you in touch with help.

Association of Breastfeeding Mothers (0207 813 1481)

They will give out numbers of counsellors who are mothers at home, available for a chat.

Breastfeeding Support Network line (0870 900 8787)

Open from 9.30am till 9.30pm every day, and puts you in touch with a breastfeeding consultant.

Lactation Consultants of Great Britain (lcgb.org.uk)

Your health visitor or midwife should be able to put you in touch with a local lactation consultant, but if you would like to research your options ahead, visit this website. Lactation consultants are trained and qualified, and cost around £30 a visit.

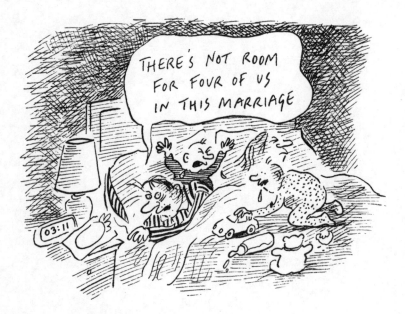

TWELVE

The Fourth Trimester

The first three months deserve their very own chapter because this is the time when you will feel that you have entered a twilight world of waking and sleeping and you exist outside the human race. Just knowing that things get easier after three months will give you a point on the calendar to look at wistfully as you sit there on the sofa feeding your babies for four solid hours while ravenously hungry yourself, with only daytime cookery programmes to keep you entertained.

Sometimes the first three months are called 'the fourth trimester' to drive home how fragile and vulnerable little newborns are, and how they would be better off still inside us. Whatever your planned approach to the fourth trimester – muddling through in your dressing gown, or maternity-nursed up to the hilt – one day around 12 weeks you will look out of the window and find yourself thinking, 'Gosh, I feel quite normal today.' Up until that moment, the real world where people get dressed and out for work by 8am will seem like this distant planet which has nothing to do with you.

Naming your babies

You may have already done this, but you may also be like many parents who have to see their newborns first before deciding what to call them. Now I know you will have been told by everyone from your doctor to the woman in the post office that it is important for the child's individuality that you don't give them names that rhyme, or start with the same letter, or that are the masculine and feminine equivalents (Ann and Andrew). What a load of tosh. Call them what you like, and if you want to call them Michael and Millie as I did, quote back that it is just as important to respect their twinship as push their different personalities.

It is no accident that some studies of identical twins, such as Louis Bouchard's Minnesota Study of Twins Reared Apart,[1] found that **identical twins separated at birth show more similar characteristics than those kept together.** Those allowed to follow their biological destiny without being artificially pushed to be more different are more similar than those who grow up in the same home. It's as if the very fact of being a twin means that there is always a struggle for individuality and identity going on from the moment of birth anyway, and this continues as the babies compete for Mummy's milk, Daddy's attention or the last piece of Marmite toast on the plate. If you want to emphasize their twinship by calling them Ned and Nancy, you can rest assured that it is unlikely to make a blind bit of difference to how they turn out.

It's far more important not to compromise, but to call them something you like the sound of, and that will roll off the tongue nicely as you shout for them to come into tea from the bottom of the garden. Identical or non-identical, they will work out their individuality for themselves.

Dressing your babies

Again, the Individuality Police have something to say about how you dress your twins. In the last few weeks of pregnancy, I read somewhere that the average twin mother spends an additional 20 minutes a day just doing up poppers on those fiddly babygros. I became obsessed by looking in second-hand shops for old-fashioned white nighties where the nappy was easily accessible. All the nighties I could find were white, and for the first few months my boy and girl twins wore nothing but white nighties.

Sure, I colour-coded their blankets and booties to help others make the distinction (but you'd be surprised how many people ask whether a baby dressed in pink is a boy), but apparently I was breaking every rule by not establishing their differences from the beginning. What a load of rubbish. I was just trying to save myself an extra few minutes, something I would suggest every twin mother does. If that means dressing them in the clothes you can reach from the baby-changing table rather than those in the tumble dryer, so be it. Just let the Individuality Police look after the babies for a few days, and see if they care what colour booties they are wearing by the end.

Sleep (for you)

It can take 12 weeks after birth for your body to 'return to normal', including important cardiovascular changes brought on by pregnancy, so don't even think about dieting or exercising in those first three months. You have only three important functions at the beginning: to eat, sleep and nurse those babies. If you are taking a career break from a good job to do this, think of the babies as your new work. And try to take a 'lunch break away from the office' at some stage in the day.

What no-one can really warn you about in the fourth trimester is **the effect of cumulative tiredness.** This isn't just one bad night, catching up the next day. It is a bad night every night with a little bit of catching up the next day. Most mothers' lowest point in the day is around 6pm or 7pm (*see introducing a one-off bottle of formula on page 175*). For other people, this is normally when the stresses of the day are over, and it's time to put your feet up. For new mothers, however, this is the time when things are just cranking up, and if you have colicky babies that start to cry at the end of the day, then you, too, might be joining them.

Every mother has a memory of The Day It All Became Too Much. Mine was handing over the baton of the babies as my husband walked in through the front door one evening. Not wanting my three-year-old to see Mummy losing it, I ran to the top of the house, slumped on the spare bed and sobbed like a heartbroken teenager. Even as the sobs were being emitted, I knew that they were tears of tiredness and toxic hormones, and had nothing to do with how wretched my life had become. And boy did I feel better afterwards. You'll have plenty of good sobs now your twins are here, just don't confuse them with wanting to divorce your husband or murder your mother-in-law. It's just cumulative tiredness, so get on the telephone to a girlfriend who will understand. Before long you will be giggling as she tells you about braining her husband with a colander at dinner when he muttered that the spaghetti wasn't cooked.

I have always maintained that the very best preparation I had for motherhood was a husband who liked to spend his (pre-baby) days out clubbing, dragging me home in the early hours of the morning. Dawn and early light became quite normal times of the day in our weekends, and occasionally watching the sun come up part of the ritual. It helped me throw away my preconceptions about how days are for doing and nights are for sleeping, and I had no idea then how grateful I would be for this rearrangement of normality. If you drop the conventional 24-hour clock thing now, it won't seem such a wrench when the babies wake at 3am. You and your body will adjust to napping and sleeping and being woken at odd times. So don't fret about what is and isn't normal.

There is only one rule to remember about sleep in those first few months, and that is the old favourite: **sleep when the babies sleep.** Even if you can't sleep, and lie there thinking about the mountain of laundry about to avalanche down the stairs, **stay horizontal**. And if you can learn to breastfeed lying on the bed, then that counts as downtime, too.

Sleep (for the babies)

I am not going to get into mentioning routines in these first few months, because I can't believe that anybody can look at a fragile newborn and want to 'train' them. Not that I wasn't under starters orders when the first few months were up, I just believe that these are precious early days so why stress yourself out by making goals that are difficult to achieve? The more you can relax into going along with the babies' needs (knowing that your own will take precedence soon enough), the less stressful life becomes.

There is one thing you can do to encourage Thing One and Thing Two to sleep: put them to sleep together in the same Moses basket or cot. I know you will have read something by the Identity Police saying that twins need to be separated, but there is plenty of time for that. These two little things have shared a womb together for nine months, so why wouldn't they want to be together? Replicating the womb experience will make them feel safe, secure and familiar, and even the movements of the other twin in their sleep will reassure rather than wake them.

Twins often share the same single pram in the early days, and there is no sweeter sight on earth. Be sure you take a few photos of them nuzzled in together, because it is all over so fast. You may even find, as I used to, one twin with a small love bite on his bald pate where the other had woken up and started to breastfeed on his head. Aaaahhhh.

Once you have got them to sleep together, you might want to get in the habit of waking them at similar times, depending on how you are feeding them. If you are breastfeeding sequentially, then you may want to feed one, wind her (or preferably give her to someone else to wind) and wake the other. If you are feeding them together by breast or bottle, they can be woken together. Although waking a sleeping baby is the most counter-intuitive thing in the world, it is never worth letting the other sleeping baby lie. If you don't do it – particularly in the middle of the night – you will either lie awake waiting for the other to wake up, or at the moment when you finally drift off, those chilling mewling sounds will start to come from the other side of the basket.

Feeding sequentially in the early days, I would have both babies in the double bed with me (they never started off there, but somehow that is where the morning found us) and breastfeed one lying down, and then walk around the bed to lie on my other side to feed the other. It seemed like a good idea at the time, until one night I stubbed my toe on the bed stumbling around in the early hours, and hopped screaming around the room.

Sex after birth

This will be the shortest section in the book. However, against all feminist better judgment, I will say the unsayable

– that **I think it is a good idea to get back into the saddle as soon as possible.** Of course, you have to feel a little bit ready for it (and the stitches brigade may think that this is sometime in a the year 3000), but as my friend Emma put it so succinctly: 'Even a blow job never goes amiss.' Or if you want nothing other than chocolate cake to pass your lips after putting up with the indignity of birth, you could always substitute a hand job for a blow job. Just remember to look sincere.

I am not thinking of you here, because I know that you do not feel like it, and that sex is somewhere low on the priority list after sleep. I am thinking of your husband or partner. Poor man. He had his wife invaded by the bodysnatchers for nine months (and in those last few months, he did his best to still fancy you); then the babies came along and he became invisible to your attentions (unless you needed him to fetch baby wipes); and finally he has been kicked out of his bed (or he can't reach you if he is still hanging in there). Throw the man a lifeline. Let him believe that there is a light at the end of the tunnel, life after birth.

A blow job will also stand you in good stead a few months down the line when cumulative tiredness makes you argue about your lack of sex life. You can point a finger at this one incident (if you never manage to repeat it) and say, 'Well most couples don't get around to doing it until a year after the birth, so at least we managed *that* after a few weeks.' This will go down a lot better than, 'For goodness sake, after a day of the babies chomping on my chest, why would I want you anywhere near me!'

Even though you may feel your libido has gone off the rails for a while, it is not necessarily a good idea to share this with your dear partner. Paying lip service, if you'll forgive the pun, is not a crime. It would be a far worse crime for your partner to believe it is him you don't fancy, not *it*.

Although it may feel as though you are going through the motions, it will be keeping you limbered up for the time when your libido returns. This may happen with a vengeance when your babies are around nine months old and stop looking teeny-weeny, and you want even tinier ones to replace them (against every practical bone in your body). 'Frankly, for the first year after each birth, I've done it to keep my husband happy rather than any desire on my part,' says one twin mum. 'I think we always put men being grumpy down to the demands of children, but mine is noticeably less grumpy after a bonk, for the next few days at least.' So don't give up on the Madonna image, now that you have taken up the Madonna and child look. You could be doing yourself a favour too, with a happier partner offering to do a few night feeds.

If you really can't face any action for a while, and have an understanding man who seems genuinely happy to wait, then you will not be alone. Talking to two twin mothers in confidence, one admitted it took two months before the subject was raised, as it were, and the other said it was closer to three months. Both had other children so their window of opportunity was limited even further by an extra guest hopping into bed with them at inappropriate moments. But both cited a desire for sleep over sex, or even having some time to themselves rather than servicing their males.

All of this may sound old-fashioned in these days of *Sex and the City*, but more modern answers are at hand as the children get older. To snatch a Saturday morning with her husband, one twin mother admitted to bribing her eldest with 50 pence to get breakfast for her twin girls. Cheap at the price.

Smiling (you and your babies)

If three months is the magic marker when life seems to get easier, there is another milestone when the whole mother-hood business gets a boost. Between two and three months, babies start to smile. This might be waved away by grannies as 'wind', but you don't care. You have sweated blood and tears to get to this two-month mark, and the smile is like a blast of sunshine in your snowy existence. You've earned it, and never has such a small smile meant so much to such a tired mother. Smiles are worth a hundred colicky moments in a mother's book, and when they happen, the room lights up.

Mark down Six Weeks on your calendar with the word SMILE. Even if you forget what it means, it might prompt you to do the same.

Crying (babies)

Because everything in early motherhood is magnified by hormones and tiredness, the sound of your babies' cries will course through your body like a pneumatic drill on your skull. You will not be able to ignore them in those first few months (later, as the babies reach their first year, you will be able to have a full conversation on the phone about British entry into the ERM without noticing both twins screeching in the background). But, for now, nature has built in a special early-warning device so that their needs are always met. Because you and the babies are still as one, the invisible umbilical cord is still there and cannot be ignored. Indeed, as a mother, from now on you will have to stop yourself from running up to every pram to comfort someone else's crying baby.

But the problem with twins is who do you go to first? And how can you settle one when the other is just starting up? There is no easy way. I used to wear one twin as an epaulette over my shoulder, holding on with one hand, while trying to plug the other twin onto my breast for a feed. Sometimes it worked, sometimes it didn't. I also used to wind one over my arm while rocking the other in a swing chair (*see Chapter 4*). These magical devices will transport you between gratitude for keeping the baby quiet and murderous rage at the dreadful tinkly music they play. Sometimes they work, sometimes they don't.

Other personal efforts to stop my babies from crying in the early days included playing my favourite tune (one that I danced around the sitting room to in my pregnancy so it had added womb-music factor) and holding them both in a cradling position as I waltzed around the table. The louder the music, the more difficult it is to hear the wails and the better chance you have of settling them. Don't worry about dropping the babies. You won't, because you are their mother.

Because I am probably not being in the least bit reassuring at this moment in time, and you are probably wondering if you can put your twins up for adoption while they are still in utero, I will hand you over to someone who really knows what he is talking about, Dr Harvey Karp. Karp believes that he has found the 'crying reflex' and a way of stopping a baby crying by turning off this crying reflex. His methods will calm even the most fretful, colicky baby in those early days. Be sure to visit his website (www.thehappiestbaby.com) or watch the video or DVD of him in action. It really has to be seen to be believed. For those who prefer a less Californian approach, there is also CRY-SIS, a national support group for parents of crying babies on 0207 404 5011.

The baby calmer

Dr Harvey Karp is a Californian professor of paediatrics at the UCLA School of Medicine and has a private practice in Santa Monica. In July 2002, Dr Karp brought out a very American book called *The Happiest Baby: The New Way to Calm Crying and Help Your Baby Sleep Longer*. I met him and his wife to discuss his methods, and am now pretty convinced that they could be a big boon for twin mothers, particularly of fussy babies. They may not be for everyone, and are only suitable for the first few months. They are based on the old idea of replicating the experience of the baby in the womb where your baby was safe, protected and nourished.

If the twins are your first babies, then the noise of them crying will at times drive you running to the bottom of the garden. Even if they are not the first, you will occasionally need to shut the bedroom door and collapse on the bed with your hands over your ears for a few minutes (Dr Karp reports that a crying baby can peak at 100 decibels, just under the noise of a chainsaw at 110).

Crying can be a big problem with twins. Even the most good-natured mother can be pushed to distraction after a couple of bad nights. But help is at hand. Karp maintains his method is 100-per-cent successful – as long as you do it right. He claims to have calmed 5,000 babies over his 20 years as a paediatrician. Michelle Pfeiffer gushes on the cover of his book, 'What every mother needs are the simple tools that really work . . . and Harvey's do.' Here is a potted version of his methods.

First, Karp says that by imitating the state of their comfy life in the womb, you will keep fussy babies happy. Before trying his technique you need to tick off that they are not hungry, wet or need winding. One box you do not need to tick because you have twins is that the babies are lonely. Some mothers even assert that their twins cried *less* than their singleton babies because they always awoke and found someone else there.

Once you have established that the babies are not crying because of their basic needs, Karp suggests the following technique to stop them crying. This is a switch he calls the 'calming reflex', which exists alongside the other 70 reflexes babies are born with, including sucking and crying.

The technique is based around the **five S's**. First **swaddle** the baby. Any midwife or granny can show you how to do this – those flannel cot sheets or pashmina scarves are good – and the trick is to do it tightly. You also have to keep babies' arms down by their sides so they don't loosen their swaddle. Swaddling a baby might seem a little unnatural at first, but remember that it has been done in all cultures for centuries, and also how tightly packed they were recently in your body. The swaddle also helps your baby to sleep longer. Karp estimates that a correctly swaddled baby will sleep at least an extra hour every day, although you need to check them to make sure that they don't get too hot. When I asked a friend whose son had been sleeping for only one hour between feeds to try swaddling, she reported back that baby Lucas slept four straight hours until waking with a wet nappy and blanket. So it worked for her.

Secondly, put the babies onto their **side** or **stomach**, which is more comfortable generally than their back. But, in keeping with current thinking about sudden infant death syndrome (cot death) and our own Back to Sleep campaign, Karp reminds us that they shouldn't be allowed to sleep on their stomachs. Once they settle or are asleep, they can be put onto their backs.

Thirdly, and this is where we get into the realms of weirdness, make very loud **shushing** noises near their ears. Apparently the sound of the mother's blood whooshing around the babies' ears in the womb is louder than a vacuum cleaner. So this shushing is supposed to be done LOUDLY. If the baby hasn't suddenly gone quiet already, it is then time to start **swinging**. This is less swinging and more a shivering movement or jiggling. The more intense the crying, the more intense the jiggling, which should settle into something more rhythmic, cool and jazz-like as the babies start to settle. You should never jiggle a baby when you are angry or upset.

Finally, there is the ultimate S – **sucking**. If, like me, you hate dummies, but still ended up buying a couple of cherry-teat soothers after a few days, you might not want to read this. But Karp insists, 'It takes a baby that is beginning to quiet and lulls him into a profound state of tranquillity . . . It triggers his calming reflex and releases natural chemicals within his brain, which leads in minutes to a rich and satisfying level of relaxation.' Mmmmm. Worth a try, no?

Like Gina Ford in *The Contented Little Baby Book*, Karp recommends whipping out the dummy and giving the baby a little jiggle once they are asleep. This teaches them to settle themselves and not become dependent on the dummy. It's a good idea because I can't tell you how many wasted hours I spent on my hands and knees under the cot searching for a bit of plastic that had fallen out and woken the baby up.

Finally, when doing the five S's, you have to add the final magic ingredients – vim and vigour. This, apparently, is why, ahem, men are so good at calming babies. Or, as Karp writes, 'the more frantically a baby is crying, the tighter his swaddling, the louder the shushing, and the more jiggly the swinging must be, or *else they simply won't work.*'

So there you have it. If you are reading this while pregnant, you are probably wondering whether you have hit upon a strange religious cult. But the alternatives are no less kooky. Our first-born, Humphrey, was a fussy baby and my husband used to zoom him around the house on his upturned forearm, his head nestled into the palm of his hand, pretending he was an aeroplane. Little did he know that he was employing three of the S techniques: shushing (or zzing), swinging and side/stomach. Another friend of mine, living in the city, used to hail a cab and jump in with a car seat when the baby started crying, because cars seem to lull small babies to sleep (all that shushing and jiggling). Cheaper to buy the book, *The Happiest Baby* at £9.99 from Amazon.

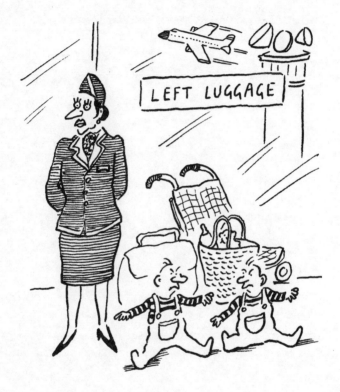

THIRTEEN

Milestones in the First Year

After those first few months, when your babies seem to emerge like butterflies from these vulnerable little chrysalises and become chubby paid-up members of the human race, you may want to reclaim a tiny bit of your life. I'm not suggesting a whole new wardrobe from Top Shop, just putting forward the concept of 'lunch' or 'tea' or 'bed-time'.

It may be that a request for some normality comes not from yourself but from your partner. Or you may have patiently given over every ounce of yourself to your newborns, accepting that your own needs played second fiddle to everyone else in the family, and now you are ready to be remembered. Wherever you stand, three months is a milestone. If you want to put off your return to real life until six months, to let the breastfeeding get established, or even for a year because you work for some Danish company (who give a year as standard maternity leave nowadays), then I hope you relax and enjoy it. And, although some days you may feel like you are stuck in an endless replay of *Groundhog Day*, with washing machines whirring and microwaves pinging, it will seem like a special time when you look back at the pictures.

If, however, you have to go back to work or get your babies into a routine IMMEDIATELY because the chaos is driving you to drink and distraction, there are plenty of rules to be had. And mostly they come from Auntie Gina, or Gina Ford of *The Contented Little Baby Book.*

The first proper night's sleep

I was introduced to *The Contented Little Baby Book* by Fiona Downes in the twins club, who had achieved the seemingly impossible after three months – making both her boys, George and Daniel, sleep through the night. Before Fiona, the babies seemed to take it in turns to sleep and eat, leaving the time in between for crying, and meals round mine were something my husband bought on the way back from the office.

But Gina changed all that. With a Nanny-Knows-Best voice, and a Scottish approach that somehow leapt off the page, she urged me to undertake her routine. She insisted that my babies be up, dressed, with their 'creases creamed' by 7am. Scared? I was.

In return for her utterly inflexible routine, you get a little bit of your life back. Routines give you some predictability for how your days will go. If you know that the babies will be 'sleeping' (in their cots with black-out blinds down, the curtains drawn and the door closed) between 12.30pm and 2.30pm, you can invite someone over for lunch. If you know that the babies should 'go down' for the night at 7pm and not need to be woken for another bottle until 10.30pm, you can organize a baby-sitter and go out to the cinema.

Because there is no easy approach to parenting – it is all about trying to do better tomorrow – there are downsides to Gina's routines. Their inflexibility means that if you want to drag the twins over to a friend's house at lunchtime, and it is supposed to be their nap time, they will be grotty and whiny as you pick over your salad. There is also a nagging sense that they have a deeply boring life, always climbing the stairs at 8.55am precisely for their morning nap. But don't be too downhearted as you abandon your Bohemian ways for a life of cast-iron predictability. Children do seem to thrive on routine in their early years, because life is so endlessly fascinating for them anyway. On balance, a routine for twins is a lifesaver for most mothers. Getting the twins to believe the same, however, takes a little time.

Establishing a routine

It took me a week of hell to make the seemingly impossible happen, to teach the babies that I would not come running with a breast or bottle every time they whimpered, nor would I pick them up until their nap time was finished. After a week, the evening came and instead of looking at my husband with a twin over his shoulder, I was staring in silence at the man whom I married a century ago. We were officially having our first evening when the babies had 'gone down' for the evening (or at least until the 10.30pm feed). Be warned.

You may find at this moment that you are not yet ready to talk to your partner. You have nothing interesting to say.

In that first week of training the babies, you need to develop an iron will and a belief that this is what you want. It may be that you are returning to work, and it would benefit everyone if you were able to write down instructions for babies' eating and sleeping habits for the incoming nanny (who wouldn't take the job without them). It may be that you just want to steal some time for yourself to sit down and read the paper in the day. Or perhaps the rest of your family would like a look-in from Mum, or a meal on the table. Whatever your reasons for wanting it, pin them to the fridge. There will be times that test your resolve and your marriage – in particular, waking sleeping babies.

There is also the small matter of breastfeeding. While it states in a matter-of-fact way in the book: 'offer the baby the right breast' or 'offer the baby the left breast to top up', breast-feeding does not sit easily with such military orders. Anecdotally, mothers have even complained of their milk supply beginning to dry up when they put their babies on Gina's routines. Certainly the routines work well for bottle-fed babies, where their food is measured out in spoons, but breast-feeding is not such a precise science. If you are breastfeeding and want to put the babies on a routine, consider using the book as a guide instead of slavishly adhering to every diktat. The general gist of the book – try to keep the babies awake as much as possible in the day when you are awake, and try to feed them as much as possible during the day so they don't want feeding in the night – is surprisingly simple. Don't feel you have to jeopardize the breastfeeding for the sake of the routine.

But for all the heartache of getting your twins to bend to Gina's ways in the early days, you are rewarded with small pockets in the day when both babies go down to sleep (the 9am to 9.30am nap was my only window for getting dressed). You will also know when they are crying because they are hungry. It is quite astonishing, really, how well it does work, and how the babies soon learn to wake up on the dot of 10.30pm for their evening bottle. It gives one a semblance of control. Until one or both of them gets a cold or starts teething. Then it's routine shmoutine, out the window.

Weaning your babies

There is a lot to be said for taking weaning seriously. Research done by Gillian Harris at Birmingham University on four-month-old babies suggests that there is a crucial eight-week window during which you can introduce curry and cabbage to avoid years of dishing up only pizza. The researchers gave four-month-old babies a teaspoon of sweet, sour, bitter and salty foods over 14 days. The test showed that babies had a preference for the foods they were exposed to over that period of time – even at the age of one. The so-called 'exposure effect' shows the importance of introducing all foods early – especially when children narrow their eating habits again at 18 months. Breastfed babies will experience many different tastes in the breast milk, so this research is particularly relevant to bottle-fed children. **The World Health Organization has recently pronounced that breastfed babies do not need to be weaned before six months**. It is less clear exactly when bottle-fed babies should be weaned (mothers of really hungry babies often start offering little bits of cereal at around 12 weeks), but four months tends to be the most common starting point.

My own limited experience proves the truth in these findings from Birmingham University. My five-year-old is a sadly typical example of British children, addicted to chicken nuggets and burgers (but a keen eater of fruit, thank heavens). His weaning was left as much to the Spanish au pair and her penchant for sugar as any insistence from me on boiling carrots. I am now convinced that my easygoing approach in the early days (especially when it came to the packet mush from supermarkets) has played a part in his poor vocabulary of foods. Don't let anyone else take responsibility for those early mouthfuls. At least if it all goes wrong later, you can look back on those first foods knowing that you did your very best.

With the twins, those hours spent spooning in parsnip purées, sticking to the letter of modern thinking, which suggests introducing one vegetable or fruit over a three-day period to test whether the babies have any allergic reactions to the food, has paid huge dividends. Now two years old, they will eat up spoonfuls of vegetables served as a side dish, and their favourite meal is cauliflower toasted in herby breadcrumbs. How much time, effort and self-flagellation I might have saved in the long run, if only I had coaxed my elder son in the early days.

As we go to print, the best weaning tables available to buy are devised by Annabel Karmel in her bestseller *The Complete Baby and Toddler Meal Planner*. Why I like Annabel Karmel over the others is that she does not insist on organic every step of the way (I tried to carry out one day's meal planner from another book – *Superfoods for Children* – and the organic produce came to £36). She also cunningly encourages children to try different tastes and textures by mixing sweet and sour. Her broccoli and pear mixture has launched a thousand tastebuds, while her ice cubes of food mush grace the freezers of mothers in castles and council estates around the UK.

The first holiday

The word 'holiday' will never sound the same again with children around. A truer phrase would be 'same work, different location' (or '*more* work' because you panic if the Sudocrem is missing from the baby change table these days). Nevertheless, we all need a change of scene sometimes, especially if you are stuck at home 24 hours a day, 7 days a week. The best way to approach a holiday is to plan the basics like a Napoleonic campaign. Just the packing alone will include two travel cots, one sterilizer, two high chairs, a stair gate for toddlers, nappies, suitcase and the changing bag.

But, for those who want to pick up Olympic medals for stressful parenting, taking baby twins abroad is the real test. We have a leaflet in the twins club library called 'Travelling with Multiples' in which two brave mothers recount their holiday horror stories of being delayed at the airport without nappies, food or milk. It is not for relaxing reading.

If you are planning to travel with your twins, think about waiting until you can afford a scheduled, rather than charter, flight. Scheduled airlines do at least offer accommodation and meal tickets if delayed, as well as carrying emergency supplies (like nappies) on board. Finally, do call ahead to the airlines and ask whether you can pre-book your seats so that your family sits together and to ask about any special aircraft safety rules. On our trip to Spain, for example, the two babies had to sit either side of the aisle because of some oxygen-mask regulation (one adult per baby per row). No small matter if you are travelling solo. On a long-haul flight, one twin mother en route to New Zealand on her own discovered that sky cots were only situated next to each other over the bulk head. She had checked in early to secure them both, fortunately.

I lost my own travel virginity when the twins were 16 months old. I was on a package holiday to Spain with my mother, and all our baby packing added up to excess baggage weighing 26kg – an extra £100 at check-in. Remember, those two little funsters get no baggage allowance at all if they are under two, which, of course, is when you most need it.

So in addition to my warning of expensive baggage habits, here are some other dos and don'ts collected from intrepid twin mothers:

1. Cut the babies' fingernails before flying out so you don't jiggle a bundle on your knee for three hours and get a scratched neck for the pleasure.
2. Always carry a big bottle of water with you, or risk paying heavily on the plane – if they carry it. It can also come in useful for washing out bottle teats should you be delayed.

3. As well as wet wipes, take a wet flannel in a plastic bag. It means babies can lick their fingers without tasting chemicals.

4. As well as a favourite cuddly toy and blanket, take a constant supply of raisins, rice cakes and organic snacks, saving some in a plastic bag for the way back. Sugary drinks and chocolate are always available, but healthy tit-bits will save on the sugar-fuelled tantrums. Just the conjuror's trick of producing something new out of the bag will also waste a few minutes on a boring flight.

5. If you are two adults travelling together, take two single buggies rather than a double buggy. Foreign pavements are often not wide enough or smooth enough for a double buggy.

6. Remember that while you may be able to zip up to the plane gate with the buggy on the way there, when you get out the other end it is likely to be a long walk to the carousel without the pushchair. Take reins to help keep toddlers upright or insist loudly on bringing your buggy into the plane (can be done despite claims of aircraft regulations).

7. Check your baby alarm and battery needs before you go. Having disposed of the plug-in leads in favour of AAA batteries, I discovered my baby alarm needed AAA rechargeable batteries, and it soon conked out after a couple of days. I would have been better off buying two converters and taking the leads.

8. Take some string as a washing line for apartment balconies. The extra washing never stops (but does at least dry quickly in hotter climates).

9. Try and get your children used to wearing sunhats before you go.

10. Consider buying wet suits for toddlers not used to swimming. The temperature difference between the hot sun and the cold pool can put toddlers off swimming altogether. T-shirt-style wetsuits, available in most catalogues, also solve the problem of constantly applying thick suntan lotion.
11. Take a throwaway camera. Even though you might be on the point of exhaustion throughout the trip, mainlining Nurofen after the transfer to the hotel, the holiday pictures will show your twins looking unbelievably cute with their pudgy arms and cheeks, and haggard Mum will be behind the camera.

I do know two friends who have resorted to Vallergan Forte, knockout drops for babies, that can only be got on prescription from a doctor who sympathizes with 'your need to help them over jet-lag'. Drugging your children is obviously the last resort for the desperate, because it does carry its own dangers. My friend administered the first spoon of Vallergan on the plane back from a Caribbean trip, and was rather horrified when both her children slept not only through the transfer at Miami, but also after the plane had landed and they had been placed in the car. They woke up a few miles from their front door in West Sussex. The drug had proved a little too effective, and although she does report it to be the easiest journey she has ever made with them, she worried that they might never wake up.

My own experience of trying to administer a spoonful to my first child en route to America threw up an altogether different response. As well as making your child unnaturally sleepy, Vallergan Forte can also have the opposite effect in a few children. It makes them hyper. After nine hours of a monstrous toddler using our thighs and the seat trays as trampolines, I can report back that our eldest son is one of those rare children. For that reason, if you do decide to do it, it is always worth trying it out *before* taking the trip.

The first sniffles and sneezes

For the record, Calpol, containing paracetamol, is the only 'drug' that can be given to babies and children under a year. In extreme cases, a doctor might suggest baby antibiotics, but most prefer not to build a baby's resistance to antibiotics too early on. **Calpol is for pain relief and does not make a child drowsy,** so there is no point dishing it out at bedtime in the hope that it might help a cold-filled baby sleep. As one who has dosed a three-month-old and a six-month-old through two operations with Calpol, with the nurses checking their watches for exact four-hour intervals, it is to be respected. Don't be seduced into thinking otherwise, especially when it's so aggressively marketed in new packet and pill form, suggesting it's a lollipop for demanding children. Calpol takes exactly 15 minutes for its effects to be felt, so, if used for flying with babies, it can be timed exactly to help ears during take-off and landing.

Homeopathic remedies

Unlike conventional medicines, pills from homeopaths are perfect for treating minor illnesses from eczema to continuous colds, earaches or tummy bugs. If you don't already have a homeopath, now would be a good time to ask around for a recommendation. The other benefit of using a homeopath is that they write copious notes about your child's health and all the subtle variations – such as the colour of the mucus – of their illnesses. On subsequent visits, using these detailed notes, the homeopath would quote back at me her record of my child's health, recording patterns that help build a picture of overall wellbeing. On my last trip to the homeopath, she noted how I had visited her a year to the day with exactly the same persistent cold and ear infection. The treatments may seem like a vaccine against the firing squad but, followed to the letter, always mysteriously worked.

The homeopath's role also doubles as a therapist for a mother, as your concerns about being the last mother on the block to crack the sleeping thing and other worries all pour out. Sometimes I would be sent home with my own bag of pills, along with the children's. But always I would leave her child-friendly office feeling lighter and reassured.

The first birthday party

This is a time of real rejoicing. It is more than a milestone. The twins' first birthday is a miracle. Don't let it pass by unnoticed. Use it as an excuse to celebrate all you have achieved in bringing your baby bundles to toddlerhood. Invite the family, friends, your midwives, new playground mates, the vicar and a few little babies. Serve champagne and cottage pie, and set the video or the cameras snapping. There is no need to organize anything at this stage except a few balloons; elaborate and expensive Mr Twizzles are to be left for the future. Right now, it is *you* who deserves to be spoilt for all the hard work it has taken to arrive here, with babies one year old.

Later, when the photos are back from the chemist, take a scrapbook and stick in every photo, lock of hair, birthday card you can find in any particular order. Forget the wedding photos and your year of backpacking around India; this album will be the most well-thumbed of all those on the bookshelf as your babies grow bigger.

Your twins are a miracle. Enjoy them while they are still yours.

References

Chapter 2

1   Figures on birth for England and Wales in 2000 from the Office of National Statistics.

2   Tuesday 15 January 2002, *The Times*, page 11.

3   Figures taken from the *Daily Mail*, Tuesday 9 July 2002 and the *Observer* 'review' page, 14 July 2002.

Chapter 3

1   P43 of *Twins! Pregnancy, Birth and the First Year of Life*, Quill, HarperCollins, 1997.

2   'Weight Gain in Twin Pregnancies' in *Nutrition During Pregnancy*, Institute of Medicine, Washington DC, National Academy Press, 1990.

3 *Everything You Need to Know to Have a Healthy Twin Pregnancy*, Gila Leiter, Dell Trade Paperback; *Twins and Multiple Births* by Dr Carol Cooper, Vermillion, 1997.

4 *Raising Multiple Children*, William and Sheila Laut, Chandler House Press, 1999, page 6.

5 *Everything You Need to Know to Have a Healthy Twin Pregnancy*, Gila Leiter, Dell Trade Paperback, page 84.

6 *Epidemiology*, quoted in *Observer Magazine*, 21 July 2002.

7 *I Don't Know How She Does It*, Allison Pearson, Chatto and Windus, 2002.

8 *Two at a Time*, Jane Seymour, Pocket Books, a division of Simon & Schuster, Inc, New York, April 2001.

Chapter 6

1 Research by Lynch & Berkowitz, New York, 1995. ('The natural history of grand multi-fetal pregnancies and the effect of pregnancy reduction').

2 *The Art of Parenting Twins*, Patricia Maxwell Malmstrom and Janet Poland, Ballantine Books, New York, 1999.

3 *Time* magazine, 10 March 2003.

Chapter 7

1 *Changing Childbirth*, edited by Beverley Beech from the Association of Improvement in Maternity Services, 1993.

2 Research shows that there is no need for this rush in uncomplicated births: Feng, Swindle and Huddleston, 1995, *Journal of Maternal-foetal Investigation*, 5, 4, 222–225; Bartnicki, Metenburg and Saling, 1992, paper on time interval in twin delivery – the second twin need not always be born shortly after the first, *Gynaecologic Obstetric Investigation*, 33, 1, 19–20.

Chapter 8

1 Common Knowledge Trust, a New Zealand outfit that sells 'The Pink Kit' and can be visited on the internet at www.commonknowledgetrust.com.

Chapter 12

1 Taken from *The Art of Parenting Twins* by Patricia Maxwell Malmstrom and Janet Poland, page 136.

Further Reading

This is where I get to show off how big my library is, thanks to my job as twins club librarian. The list of books below is not comprehensive, but it is up to date, and all of the following can be bought from Amazon.com at the time of going to press. All the new twin books are American, which means the language is more Barney the Dinosaur ('I love you, you love me, we're a happy family') than Bob the Builder. You have been warned.

New twin books

***Two at a Time: Having Twins. The journey through pregnancy and birth* by Jane Seymour and Pamela Patrick Novotny (Simon & Schuster, 2001)**

Jane Seymour, the British actress who stars in the drama *Dr Quinn*, lives in America, so her experience of having twins in sunny California may not tally much with those of us holed up in a rainy Britain. Particularly surprising is her intensive workout regime during her pregnancy, listed in great detail, until her pregnancy ends abruptly with pre-eclampsia and a Caesarean at 34 weeks. Nevertheless, her story does make compulsive reading, possibly because it reads like *Hello!* magazine – as this paragraph on the subject of pumping breast milk demonstrates: 'There was an unforgettable moment in the home of a very famous, major figure in the film industry [but who, Jane who?] whose elegant wife had never had children. Poor man came home from work one evening and there I was in this extremely fancy bathroom area pumping away. I thought to myself afterwards – could that be why I've never seen those people since? At the very least, he probably never again thought of me as a glamorous actress!' Pass the breast milk bag.

Twin Tales: The Magic and Mystery of Multiple Birth by Donna M. Jackson (Little Brown, 2001)

This is mainly a photographic book with some utterly adorable pictures of twins, identical and otherwise. There is little text (good for those with short attention spans) and some fantastic pub-bore information on the more unusual issues – conjoined twins, twin telepathy, 'super-duper' twins (the Chukwu Octuplets, McCaughey Septuplets and the Thompson Sextuplets). For a coffee-table read, this is a great book, because it also documents the odd serious issue, such as the experiments carried out on 3,000 twins who passed through Dr Mengele's laboratory in Auschwitz.

***The Joy of Twins and other Multiple Births: Having, raising and loving babies who arrive in groups* by Pamela Patrick Novotny (Three Rivers Press, 1994)**

Although the author promises us the 'joy', this book quickly falls into line with many others and focuses on all the problems and depression that often beset us mothers of multiples. Headings such as 'How can I feel such loss when I have been given so much?' sum it up. Nevertheless, this is a well-thought out book with a good chapter on breastfeeding, as well as lots of psychological stuff on twin bonding and separating twins later. And for those feeling a little overwhelmed by it all, you can always turn to the chapter on 'What is Good About Having Twins' and learn that twins are more confident, supportive, self-knowing, innovative, sought-after and (ahem) giving. The only slight disappointment was that this chapter is only four pages long.

***Raising Multiple Birth Children. A parents' survival guide* by William and Sheila Laut (Chandler House Press, 1999)**

This is one of the few books written by triplet parents, so should be snapped up just for the fun of it by any triplet (heroine) mothers out there. It is filled with exclamation marks, a busy layout and Americanisms, but is relentlessly good-humoured (as all triplet mothers have to be, presumably). The American shopping list is fascinating (what is 'The Boss' LITE Cordless Sweeper by Eureka on the must-have checklist?), although sadly the list of free products from Wal-Mart and Fisher-Price will not extend to Old Blighty.

Twins! Pregnancy, Birth and the First Year of Life by **Connie L. Agnew, MD, Alan H. Klein and Jill Alison Ganon (HarperCollins, 1997)**

This is the only book I have ever seen which offers a monthly guide to what the babies look like in your stomach. If, like me, you liked Gordon Bourne's singleton pregnancy book because it had sketches of the babies at every week and descriptions of them being 'about the size of a banana', then this book will definitely appeal. Being American, much of the emphasis on medical care and immunization schedules will be different, but the round-table discussion format, where lots of different parents of twins interrupt each other about their experiences, works surprisingly well.

Raising Twins (From birth through adolescence) by **Eileen M. Pearlman & Jill Alison Ganon (HarperCollins 2000)**

The same author, Jill Alison Ganon, co-writes the sequel to the above, and tackles such thorny issues as teenage twins and how to separate twins into different bedrooms. Again, it's all-American advice, and I object to bossiness over what to call my children, but the round-table format with twins themselves talking about their twinship gives unexpected insights. For example, when Dr Pearlman asks Amaro whether he fights much with his fraternal twin Hermes, he answers, 'Yes, plenty. It's blood lust. We don't talk when we fight.'

Everything You Need to Know to Have a Healthy Twin Pregnancy (a doctor's step-by-step guide for parents of twins, triplets, quads and more!) by **Gila Leiter, MD (Random House, 2000)**

This is an excellent, extremely thorough guide with illustrations of the combinations of identical twins, sketches of a baby's head coming out during a Caesarean, and a list of every single drug imaginable that can or cannot be ingested during pregnancy. I would highly recommend buying this for your midwife or doctor to read, but I would hesitate reading it yourself if pregnant. It is doom-laden. Because every aspect of the High Risk pregnancy is picked over in detail by the author (a doctor and mother of twins), no aspect of care is omitted. For example, this book tells you 'if your partner likes to blow air into your vagina during sex it could lead possibly to a fatal embolism [air bubble] in your lung'. Yikes.

***The Art of Parenting Twins* by Patricia Maxwell Malmstrom and Janet Poland (Ballantine Publishing Group, 1999)**

Written by the former chair of Twin Services Inc. for 20 years, this has plenty of anecdotes collected over her time and good advice for the clueless newcomer. It also goes all the way up to adolescence and adulthood, with some milestone chapters in between, such as 'Toddler Dilemmas and Delights: Your Twins, ages one to three'. Apart from being a little repetitive and wordy, it can't be faulted as an overall glimpse of the road ahead.

Old faves

***Having Twins* by Elizabeth Noble (Houghton Mifflin, 1991)**

Despite its date of publication and its very American-ness, I still feel this is the best handbook ever written on the subject. It is particularly good on the pregnancy and birth stuff – sadly there is precious little for the reader who has already got two healthy babes. Few other books tackle chapters so confidently on all the tricky subjects.

The Twins Handbook by Elizabeth Friedrich and Cherry Rowland (Robson Books, 1984)

This has been standard fare for many years. I found it dry and boring, but it does cover all the facts.

Twins, Triplets and More by Elizabeth M. Bryan (Penguin, 1992)

See above, with a bit more history and a section on twin death and the surviving twin. Not uplifting stuff and a little scanty on the newborn period and first year.

Twins & Multiple Births: The Essential Parenting Guide from Birth to Adulthood by Dr Carol Cooper (Vermilion, 1997)

I found this dry and unappealing, although it does cover all the basics without any partisan preference to, say, natural birth versus Caesareans, and it does go all the way up to secondary school. Don't be fooled by the cartoon on the front – there are no jokes in here.

Not about twins, but worth reading...

The Best Friend's Guide to Pregnancy by **Vicki Iovine (Bloomsbury, 1997)**

I was sent this book by a pregnant friend in America, and promptly burnt all the other pregnancy bibles on a roaring fire. It documents the path to motherhood with wit and laugh-out-loud humour, and tackles the difficult subjects such as sex and why you suddenly hate your partner. Vicki Iovine deserves the American equivalent of an OBE for services to womankind for writing this book.

The New Contented Little Baby Book by **Gina Ford (Vermilion, 2002)**

The bible for twin mothers in search of a good routine. Prepare to pinch salt and adapt for the twin factor.

How Not to be a Perfect Mother by **Libby Purves (HarperCollins, 1986)**

A right rollicking read from my favourite journalist and Radio 4 presenter who will knock you flat with her good sense and wise words. If you can't face any of the others, just buy this.

How to be a Pregnant Father by **Peter Mayle (Citadel Press, 1986)**

Before he wrote *A Year in Provence*, Mayle was doing the words for this illustrated survival guide for the father-to-be. It might be something to put under the nose of a partner fed up with fetching avocado sandwiches for you, particularly as it includes a few basic recipes. Funny illustrations and no bearded 1970s casualties in sight.

Siblings without Rivalry by Faber and Mazlish (Piccadilly Press, 1999)

A very American tale of a Sibling Without Rivalry Workshop Group, and the first-person experiences of those within it. Good for anyone anxious about new babies upsetting the sibling status quo.

Birth over 35 by Sheila Kitzinger (Sheldon Press, 1994)

Good, comprehensive and partisan stuff from the high priestess of natural birth, although it is a little political for most. A good antidote for anyone fed up with being labelled as 'high risk' by doctors. Sheila also spares us the other people's birth photos in this book.

Solve your Child's Sleep Problems by Dr Richard Ferber (Dorling Kindersley, 1986)

This is detailed, technical and reassuring with lots of different sleep problems outlined. Worth buying or borrowing before you have twins because, if you need it, you will be far too tired to buy it and read it afterwards. Ferber's controlled crying technique gives you a precisely timed routine to help your children fall asleep on their own.

Index